My Mother's Keeper

A Middle-Aged Son's Experiences
As Caregiver For
His Alzheimer-Afflicted Mother

Bob Apperson

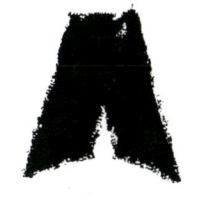

Authority Press Inc.

© 2001 Authority Press Inc.
All rights reserved. Published by Authority Press Inc. No part of this book may be reproduced in any form without written permission from the Publisher. The views and concepts presented are those of the contributors. Publication by Authority Press Inc. does not in any way constitute endorsement or approval of the book's contents. No responsibility is assumed by the Publisher for any injury and/or damage to persons or property as a matter of product's liability, due to negligence or otherwise, or from any use or operation of any methods, products, instructions, or ideas contained in the material herein.

Printed in the United States of America.

04   03   02   01   1   2   3   4   5

Authority Press Inc.
10970 Morton's Crossing
Alpharetta, GA 30022
770-475-2837
www.authoritypress.com

Publisher: Eric E. Torrey
Editor: Elizabeth Gordon
Cover: Craig Hall, Streambed Graphics
Printed by: QUESTprint

Table of Contents

Chapter One, Page 1
Welcome To My World... An Introduction
The purpose of this book is to give you, the medical layman, a view from the eyes of another layman of what you might (or might not) expect if you are thrown in the path of this fast-moving train.

Chapter Two, Page 5
Hello Mother... I'm Your Son
Nobody will ever know how many nights I silently wept and wondered what I had done to be given this ultimate test.

Chapter Three, Page 13
Living With The Three-Minute Window
Short-term memory gets shorter and shorter. Caregivers must devise methods that help them deal with the window.

Chapter Four, Page 21
Avoiding A Trip To Bonkersville!
If you become someone's caregiver, you must think of your well-being as much as the well-being of the person for whom you have assumed responsibility.

Chapter Five, Page 29
Please Don't Pull The Patch Off!
This period was a terrific indoctrination for what lay ahead. Every day brought a new challenge to overcome.

Chapter Six, Page 35
How Many More Stale Cheese Sandwiches Will I Find?
Every case has its own characteristics with some similarites, so there are no hard-and-fast guidelines. Caregivers have to play-it-by-ear and develop their own guidelines.

Chapter Seven, Page 41
I Wonder What's In The Attic... Besides Mother!
There are certain things that you must do, whether you want to or not. It comes with the territory.

Chapter Eight, Page 47
Come Help Me Burn The House Down!
You never know what will happen next, so a caregiver has to be alert to everything.

Chapter Nine, Page 53
Doctor, Doctor... Please Spare Me The Pain
I would like to point out that the caregiver's health is as important as the health of the one being attended. I can speak from experience.

Chapter Ten, Page 59
A Very Puzzling Thing
Mother couldn't remember who had visited or what she had eaten, but she could remember words and their meanings with no problem. It amazed me!

Chapter Eleven, Page 63
Tell Me That Story Again, Mother... And Again... And Again...
Even when Mother's stories would get confused, she still told them as if she knew that every word was correct.

Chapter Twelve, Page 69
Something's Wrong With The Furnace
You have to do what you think is best regardless of what people think. You are in a better position to know your finances, the needs of the person for whom you are caring, and what you need personally.

Chapter Thirteen, Page 77
Padlock The Freezer Door And Out With The Kitchen Cabinet Shelves
You have to learn to cope. I developed patience by ignoring things that I could not control. I kept telling myself that certain things really didn't matter.

Chapter Fourteen, Page 83
Grocery Bags Make A Fine Suitcase
I was always anxious at night and my sleep wasn't as restful as I needed it to be. Sleep without rest is not very useful.

Chapter Fifteen, Page 89
Would You Please Wind My Watch?
Mother was obsessed with time. She was continually looking at her watch, asking me to wind it, and asking me the time. This obsession with time is a mystery to me to this day.

Chapter Sixteen, Page 93
The Old Swith-The-Walking-Stick Trick
Mother knew that something was wrong with her memory, but really didn't understand the problem. Sometimes she would say that she wondered where she had been for years.

Chapter Seventeen, Page 97
Mentioning The Unmentionables
My relatives were a great help with the personal hygiene problems. Mother loved the attention and it was very much appreciated by me.

Chapter Eighteen, Page 101
That Dreaded Bedroom Door
Why should a bedroom door be such a problem? Because I never knew what I would find behind that door, that's why.

Chapter Nineteen, Page 105
Another Angel Has Flown
Lucile Thomason Apperson, October 3, 1905 - March 7, 1994

Appendix
Don't Take My Word For It
Some of the best references that the author was able to find.

Chapter One

Welcome To My World...
An Introduction

The purpose of this book is to give you, the medical layman, a view from the eyes of another layman of what you might (or might not) expect if you are thrown in the path of this fast-moving train.

Close your eyes. Imagine that you are a 56-year-old male with absolutely no more cooking skills than the average Tenderfoot Boy Scout. Boiling water requires a recipe! Burnt toast is an hors d'oeuvre! Imagine that your housekeeping skills are limited to changing a roll of toilet paper or getting a clean towel. Imagine that you are thrown back into a world that you left almost 40 years before and all of the landmarks are gone. You have no idea where anything is or how to even find the grocery store. Imagine that you find yourself the caregiver for an Alzheimer victim who happens to be your 84-year-old mother.

I didn't have to imagine. One day I found myself in that predicament and there was no turning back. I was an only child and this duty was falling on my watch. I had two choices: I could put Mother in a nursing home and walk away. Or I could take the bull by the horns and try to provide the comfort of her small but beloved home for her while she spent her waning moments on Earth. I chose the latter. Got gored by the bull many times as her waning moments stretched into waning months and then years. But I succeeded in achieving my goal...not flawlessly...but I let her die in her sleep in her bed in her home, and I take great pride in it. And I give my utmost thanks to all who reached out to help in so many ways. Without the help of friends and family I would have gone down in flames.

It all started with a phone call. My cousin Sarah, a nurse, called me in Florida, my home for many years, and said that Mother was having cataract operations. She said that I needed to come up to Virginia for about ten days to take care of Mother as she recuperated. She said that Mother's memory was on a downhill slope. Sarah was a prophet...except the slope was more like a dive off a cliff! When I saw her condition first-hand, I got back in my van, drove to Tampa, picked up what I could tote, and headed back to an adventure that even Mark Twain couldn't have written.

How does a guy reach the age of 56 with no cooking skills? Simple. For the first 18 years I ate my mother's excellent food. Then I spent three years eating Air Force chow hall food. Granted, that was enough to make one want to learn to cook, but stoves weren't allowed in the barracks.

My next move to avoid cooking was to marry a wonderful cook. She kept me out of the kitchen for 27 years. Then we divorced and I found a friend to live with who was another wonderful cook. Now I was faced with feeding my mother and myself, and had a lot of learning to do.

My trip to Tampa and back was filled with quandaries. Anybody who says you can't teach an old dog new tricks should find himself faced with my dilemma. It was learn to cook or starve. I love to eat...so this old dog took a crash course and soon acquired some basic skills. It turned out that basic skills were all that would be needed.

Many of you reading this will face a similar situation. Cancer used to be the most dreaded disease on Earth. But in my humble opinion it has been replaced by a plight that spreads its tentacles around everybody near and dear to the victim and renders them victims, too. What we used to refer to as senility when I was a boy has now been honored with its own familiar name and nomenclature. It cannot be mistaken for something that happens routinely to the aged and aging. I lost one of my best buddies to it while I was caring for Mother. He was only 58 when he was besieged...only 61 when he died. He didn't even know his wife before it took him away. This painful killer is Alzheimer's disease, marked by progressive loss of mental capacity resulting from degeneration of the brain cells. It was named after Alois Alzheimer, a German neurologist who lived from 1864 to 1915.

The purpose of this book is to give you, the medical layman, a view from the eyes of another layman of what you might (or might not) expect if you are thrown in the path of this fast-moving train. Maybe I should tell you to get off the tracks, but chances are you won't be able to move fast enough! In any event, I will tell you that it will not be all bad. If you have a sense of humor you'll come out with flying colors, because there will be many things to laugh at...and a fair share of times that you will bawl your eyes out. But the balance will keep you trucking! My dear mother, even though she was parked in a fog bank with her foot on the mental clutch, said many times...laughter is the best medicine.

I have tried to make this light reading. Just remember something I wrote to a business acquaintance many years ago...

Today's trauma is tomorrow's trivia!

Chapter Two

Hello Mother... I'm Your Son

*Nobody will ever know
how many nights I silently wept
and wondered what I had done
to be given this ultimate test.*

After the phone call from my cousin telling me about Mother's cataracts and other physical, I had to make plans to be gone for several weeks. The last thing I wanted to do was spend time away because I had an established routine and I am a creature of habit. Most of us are! So I postponed the trip as long as I could. Finally I couldn't stall any longer and packed a few things for a short stay. It never entered my mind that my stay would be longer than my Air Force tour of duty. Boy, was I in for a surprise! I left Tampa, Florida early in the morning and drove straight through to Mechanicsville, Virginia, just east of Richmond. It took 14 hours and I was a tired camper when I finally pulled into Mother's driveway at the house where I grew up. I was very excited about seeing Mother. It had been five long years and I expected her to be excited, too. It seemed that the older we got, the less we saw of each other. She didn't travel any more, and I had put the trip off through pure procrastination. We talked on the phone and wrote, but time passed without a visit. My daughters had visited her and told me about her forgetfulness, but I passed it off as simply old age. In the past, she had always been elated when I came to see her. On many business trips up North I would arrange a layover in Richmond so I could get some of that good old home cooking. I was an only child and my mother doted on me. I was in for another big surprise this time.

When I arrived, Mother was seated in the rocker that she had inherited from my grandfather. It was beside the radiator next the front window and would be a sight etched into my mind for life. I spent a long four years watching her sit and rock in that exact same spot. She didn't recognize me when I came into the living room. I had to tell her who I was. This was a real shock and very unsettling to me. At first I attributed her not knowing me to the cataracts. It didn't take long for me to realize that it went deeper than cataracts. My mother's mind was slipping gears.

During the last five years I had called her at least monthly just to chat and see how she was. I noticed from time to time that she was a bit forgetful, but I figured it just came with the aging process. In a recent phone call I asked if she had received flowers that I had just sent. She wasn't sure; she had to leave the phone and find the flowers. That should have been my first clue, but I guess I was in denial. My mother was an eternal being in my mind's eye. Infallible! I had to see her in person for her condition to sink in.

I now sit in that same rocker when I watch TV. From time to time it enters my mind that some day I might be rocking and looking out of the window just as Mother did. It is a sobering thought and one that you, my reader, must also consider. Until a solution to the Alzheimer's problem is discovered, we are all candidates. Little did I know that night how this disease would change my life. I think frequently of how Mother went from being the most independent person I have ever known to a childlike dependent of her only child.

After being reminded several times that I was her son, she started to get it right and was very glad to see me. She had no idea why I was there, although she had been told many times that I was coming and why I was coming. Being very naïve, I assumed it would sink in eventually and things would be like old times. This lady had contributed so much to my life and had been my greatest supporter in all of my endeavors...regardless of how hare-brained they turned out to be. To see her fog-bound was extremely depressing. It registered quickly that I had a job ahead of me and didn't know whether I was up to the challenge.

Mother toddled off to bed not long after I arrived and I sat alone and pondered my situation. I was suffering van lag, still quivering from road vibration. What was I to do? The ball was squarely in my court now. In the past I always had a hold card, regardless how bad it got. I always had my mother to fall back on for opinions, support, and even a little financial help if needed. Now I was beginning to doubt the expression "no man's an island". I felt like an island far from the shores of sanity and safety. I had some big-time planning to do and I had to do it quickly.

In 1985 I owned a display design and manufacturing company that was battling financial strain. That strain translated to stress on me. My blood pressure was higher than the national debt and I couldn't get it under control. So my doctor gave me two choices...either close the business or he would attend my funeral. I didn't like him well enough to want him at my funeral, so I opted to close the business. For several years I did just enough to get by financially and my health improved enough for me to feel fairly safe. I did have a few customers and I had to explain my situation to them and help them find another display designer. I had learned to adjust my lifestyle to fit my budget and this would help me in the years to come. Mother was living on social security and not a big monthly check at that.

When I was in the Air Force years ago, our Technical Instructor in basic training told us that all a person needed to survive in life were "three hots and a cot." Food and a place to put your head were the essentials. All the rest were material objects with little meaning. Now I was about to find out how true that statement really was. I was going to be without any income—but at least Mother did have a cot for me. In fact, she had the bed that I slept in until I left home in my late teens. Time flew as I pondered my future; I finally went to bed totally confused and dead tired. I was battling an adrenaline rush that would keep me tossing and turning for quite some time.

The next morning brought the proof I needed to force me

to make up my mind. It was just as though the previous day had never happened. I was up when Mother arose and came into the living room. I had to explain to her again who I was and why I was there. I had no idea what Alzheimer's disease was, but I was soon to find out! Mother was glad to see me after we went through the Hi, Mother…I'm your son routine again. The big problem was that she thought I was sixteen again and she had to care for me. She wanted to prepare breakfast for me, but I had to help her fix a bowl of cereal. This lady had been one of the best cooks ever and now had trouble getting milk onto a bowl of cereal!

I started gathering the facts. Mother was 84 years old. Besides cataracts she had a heart problem, high blood pressure and high cholesterol. She was in the care of a cardiologist who she had obtained when I asked my aunt and cousin to get a second opinion. The previous doctor wanted to catheterize her to check plaque buildup in the artery to her brain. He gave her a 50-50 chance of surviving the test and I immediately shouted NO! He said that plaque could break loose and block the blood flow to the brain. Eighty-four years old and undergoing a test that could end it all! I didn't believe that to be a sensible procedure and asked for another doctor who agreed with me. My conclusion was that I had better get back to Tampa and make arrangements for a prolonged stay in Virginia.

I have to give my cousin Virginia (who lived several doors from Mother), my Aunt Hazel and my cousins Sarah and David hearty thanks for their vigilance and caring attention to Mother as her mind progressively failed her. I really felt more like an outsider. These people had been involved with Mother daily while I had been 800 miles south. I felt that Mother was in good hands for the short time that I would be gone. Virginia had done Mother's shopping since she sold her car and stopped driving some five years previously. I asked her to keep an eye on Mother and I climbed into my van and made a whirlwind round-trip run.

On the way back three days later, I had another wake-up call. I called Mother when I got into Richmond to let her know that I was on my way. I was still living in the past; I hadn't become acclimated to the fact that Mother wouldn't even remember that I had been there and gone just several days before. At first it was like talking with a complete stranger.

Finally it registered with her who I was and I got a warm invitation to come visit! WOW! My mother was inviting me to visit. I had just plotted another point on the learning curve.

I returned with clothes, my small computer and printer and not much else. All that I knew was that I was bound and determined to keep my mother in her home as long as I possibly could. My father had been overcome by carbon monoxide poisoning when Mother was only 51 years old. He spent 12 years in a mental hospital. Mother had to go to work for the first time since she was forced to quit teaching when she was married. She hadn't worked outside the home since she was 22 years old. Daddy left her with a mortgaged home and other debt because he wasn't a very good businessman. This proud, determined woman went to work for my uncle at a bit above minimum wage, paid off the debts and socked away a respectable saving until she retired at age sixty-two. She loved the little home that she had paid off and I was going to do everything in my power to let her to live out her life in it.

What I had ahead of me in the coming weeks was much like starting a new business. I had to familiarize myself with Mother's financial situation, what income to expect, what her fixed monthly outlay was, her bank accounts, and any other places where money was going to come from or go. It turned out that Mother had made a very orderly arrangement for her financial setup. She lived frugally and every penny had its place! Back in 1973 when Daddy died she did something that would make my life much easier now. She put my name on everything, including the deed to the house. We were co-owners. Everything was set up with signatures signed with "or" rather than "and", so I could sign without her co-signature. This really helped because it was extremely difficult to explain to Mother what it was she was signing if she did need to sign.

I went through a very frustrating episode when I got her to grant me Power of Attorney. Although I was co-owner of everything, there were certain things that I had to have Power to execute. Mother had assigned Power of Attorney to my aunt when she first started having problems with her memory. Now I would be handling her affairs, but she couldn't understand why her child needed to take care of her business! As I said before, she thought I was still in my teens and she was caring for me. I finally got her to sign and one more challenge was overcome.

Mother became very nervous if she didn't have a checkbook in her pocketbook and a few bucks in her wallet. I finally had to remove the checkbook. If anybody knocked on the door soliciting, she would write a check and really mess things up! I had to learn all of this the hard way and learn it fast. Removing the checkbook set off another rocket. Mother would go through every drawer in her dresser searching for the darned thing and get so nervous that I thought she would have a stroke. I had to distract her long enough for her to forget what she was searching for and get her settled down. It took quite some time for her to forget that she usually had a checkbook in her pocketbook. I experienced this routine until I thought I'd go crazy. It finally ended, thank God!

My next goal was to get her in better health. Mother's cardiologist gave me a booklet of healthy diets to lower cholesterol and I put her on a regimented diet. In several months I had the cholesterol under control and kept the blood pressure down with medication. Mother loved all of the wrong things. I really felt guilty about rationing things like ice cream. At first I had to eliminate it from the grocery list until I figured out how to handle Mother's forgetful craving. She ate a half-gallon in one day before I realized what was happening. She would eat a bowl, forget that she had, then she would eat another bowl. I'll tell you in another chapter what I finally had to do to take control and be able to ration a simple thing like ice cream.

Every day brought something new with which I had to contend. My aunt had bought a pill organizer that had compartments for a week's supply of pills, three compartments a day for seven days. Before I came, she would come out weekly and fill the organizer for Mother. One morning I came into the dining room and found Mother sitting at the table with every compartment open. Her favorite expression was "they said" when she tried to explain why she was doing things. She looked up at me and told me, "They said I have to take all of these pills." She would have consumed the whole week's supply if I hadn't been there. How she made it as long as she had before I arrived is a mystery to me to this day. I'm sure that my presence was a confusion factor until she got used to my being there ...for her and me, too!

Needless to say, I swore myself in as the Pill Police Chief and kept both the medication and the pill organizer well out of sight. It became my duty to dole out medication with Mother's meals and make sure she took the pills. Many times she would ask why she was taking medicine and I came up with a canned pitch. She disliked having to go visit a doctor. Many years passed without her ever seeing one. So my pitch was simple. I would tell her that the doctor said that if she didn't take her pills we would have to go to his office. The pills went down faster than a skydiver who forgot his chute! Mother was generally docile and that made my job much easier.

Regardless of Mother's docility, I was walking through a minefield and felt so helpless. The first several months were as stressful as the business that I had to close. Here I was, a 56-year-old man thrown into the frightful task of caring for a lady who was disconnected from reality. Nobody will ever know how many nights I silently wept and wondered what I had done to be given this ultimate test. But my mother had taken care of me when I was an unknowing youngster; she had probably been faced with as many dilemmas as I would face. It was payback time. So I had to keep saying Hello Mother, I'm your son...and hope that she would finally remember.

Chapter Three

Living With The Three-Minute Window

Short-term memory gets shorter and shorter. Caregivers must devise methods that help them deal with the window.

Just what is a three-minute window? I use the phrase to describe Mother's short-term memory problem. She usually had to be reminded who people were when they visited. After they were introduced to Mother, she could hold a reasonable conversation. When they left, her memory left too. In a very short time Mother had no recollection of having had visitors, much less of who they were. It was both amusing and frustrating. Three minutes is simply a manner of speech. The time varied and every Alzheimer's victim has different symptoms; but the window is common to most, and the narrowing of the window is a signal to the caregiver. Short-term memory is still there but it gets shorter and shorter. Caregivers must devise methods that help them deal with the window.

Memory is a mysterious but wonderful thing. Some people have bad memories naturally, while others have what we call photographic memories. Since we are all unique, there is a wide range of memory ability. We have both short-term and long-term memories and each has its purpose. We work daily in short-term memory for such things as remembering telephone numbers we want to dial and what we want to do next when we're working on a project. We store important things that we want to preserve for the future in long-term memory. The interesting thing about Alzheimer's victims is that they have better long-term than short-term recall. They tend to live in the past. Mother reviewed her relatives on a continual basis and asked over and over..."is so-and-so gone?" Since her ability to remember things in the present was diminished, she couldn't store my answer, so she would ask again and again. The past remained in place since she couldn't update the information. She would say after I told her that so-and-so had passed on, "Where have in the world have I been?" Another of her expressions that became part of a continuing dialog started with the phrase, "Did I dream it, or has so-and-so passed on?" Then we would go through the same conversation one more time.

Most of my professional life has been spent in sales, marketing, and advertising. Memory plays a big part in all three endeavors. You have to make your product or service memorable to get people to buy. So I used the Ebbinghaus Memory Curve in my presentations to sell advertising and, later, displays. The good Dr. Ebbinghaus studied the rate at which we forget. He found through extensive study that the human brain forgets a great amount of what is seen, read or heard in a very short time. In fact, we retain approximately 58 percent for only 19 minutes! Then forgetfulness trails off and we retain 20 percent of the remaining information after 30 days.

Why do I tell you this in a discussion of my mother's malady? I tell you because I used the same technique to help her with her three-minute window that I used for my clients when I promoted their wares: Repetition. Repetition reinforces memory and therefore decreases forgetfulness. If you are exposed to something enough you will remember it. This is why you see the same commercial on TV over and over. If the commercial is well done, it doesn't bother you. If it is obnoxious, you want to throw something at the TV. The interesting thing is that you remember them both after enough exposures. Remember how you crammed for exams in school? You read the words, equations, formulas, or whatever you wanted to remember over and over. Usually it stuck. I knew that it worked in advertising, and found that it helped Mother retain things. As time went on it became harder and harder to overcome her problem, but for the first several years it did work enough to keep me repeating what to some might seem to be trivial.

When visitors left, I waited long enough for Mother to settle down from the stimulation of the visit. Then I would test the window. Invariably she would not remember that anybody had visited. At this point I would start giving hints and jarring her memory until she would, with a little help, start to recall. As years passed it became harder and harder to bring recall. But I kept at it until I no longer had a mother to care for and I do believe that my efforts prolonged her life.

The interesting thing about Mother was that once a visitor or visitors were engaged in conversation, she had the ability to remember such things as children's and spouse's names. She had to be told things over and over during the conversation, but I was always amazed at her ability to associate people with people. Also, for the first several years she was never left out of the conversation. Mother was, by nature, a social creature and loved interchange with people. In many ways, even though she was unconnected with reality, she never ceased to amaze me. She was a very warm, loving person and people loved her because she empathized with them. She was a favorite aunt with her nieces and nephews and their attention was very important to her. She had a way with everybody and was treated with respect even in her unwanted return to a childhood state. This attitude exhibited by others was invaluable to me in my difficult chore of caregiver.

Mother always had a delightful sense of humor. Her forgetfulness never impeded her ability to giggle at some of my absurd attempts to be funny. She said many times that her mother had told her that laughter was the best medicine. So I made little jokes about her forgetfulness and we laughed. Mother was a very religious person, although she hadn't been in church for many years. One of my favorite little word games had to do with the gospel. Instead of "only begotten son" I called myself her "only forgotten son". It always brightened her eyes and usually brought a kind rebuttal. I never criticized her for not remembering. Her three-minute window seemed to expand when we were joking and she was laughing, so I made it a point to try to tickle her funny bone as often as I could. Mother was aware that she had a problem but didn't really comprehend the problem. She couldn't remember that she couldn't remember. But she wasn't living in the real world...so it really didn't matter to her! I believe that her dis-association from reality helped extend her life. Stress is a true killer and Mother had long since left her stress behind.

There was a noticeable change in her recall during the first six to eight weeks after I came to live with her. I don't pretend to know any of the technical reasons for this improvement, but I surmise that having someone to speak with had something to do with it. Mother had lived alone for years. This was not bad until she gave up her ability to drive and became more housebound. She sat and looked...yes looked...at television hour after hour. She couldn't keep up with the story but she did like her soap operas. Although she had some visitors, she spent lots of time with no conversation. As her memory began to go, she became more and more inward. I think this was a degenerative condition that caused the memory to get worse. My arrival on the scene, having someone to say "good morning" to when she got up and "good night" to when she was ready for bed, caused her brain to become more active. Her three-minute window was swinging open. Again, this is just supposition, but I really saw a change. I had hopes at first that she really didn't have Alzheimer's Disease. Although this turned out to be untrue, it sure made my transition to caregiver much easier to handle.

Nobody knows exactly what brings on dementia. I believe that my mother's problem was directly related to a head injury. In the early 80's she had a bad fall. She was on the kitchen counter setting her wall clock. She stepped back onto her stepstool and missed. Down she went onto the floor on her head.

Mother was obstinate about certain things. One of those things was visiting doctors. My cousin Sarah was a nurse and tried to get her to see a doctor after she fell. She had a distinct knot on her head and should have had it treated. But no, Mother insisted that she was fine and didn't go. Soon her arm and hand started to go numb. Finally, after about a month, Sarah got her into the emergency room and immediately into surgery. They had to drill a hole in her skull and let the blood out that had built up between her brain and cranium. The numbness went away, but I think damage had been done that affected her memory. Soon after this happened, driving started to make Mother nervous so she decided to stop driving. A downward spiral began and her memory became worse and worse. She was in her late 70's and had a remarkable memory before the fall, so I have to attribute her problem to the injury.

Another reason is that there is evidence that the disease has genetic predisposition. To my knowledge, Mother is the only member of her immediate family that suffered the malady. Here again, I have no scientific proof...just uneducated guessing...and plenty of hope that I am right. After all, I am in that genetic chain! As an interesting aside, in just 23 generations our gene pool is derived from 4,194,304 people! That's only 529 years, if we consider a generation to be an average 23 years. So you can easily see that we are all vulnerable even though there is no evidence of the disease in known relatives.

Since I had no knowledge of the problem I was now facing, I started investigating. As I mentioned earlier, my high school buddy was besieged with the disease. I hadn't seen Harold in almost forty years and had never met his wife, Jean. I wanted to talk with her but felt that I needed someone to introduce me so I wouldn't appear to be a complete idiot. My cousin Carolyn came to the rescue. She knew someone who knew Harold's wife and arranged for me to call her. We had a good conversation by phone.

It was immediately apparent that Harold's symptoms were different in many ways from Mother's. He had no injuries or other reasons for his memory loss. He just started to get forgetful. In a very short time it had degenerated into a real problem. Jean invited me to come see him, but warned me that he probably wouldn't remember me. I took the chance anyway.

Thank God for small favors! Although I was sailing in uncharted waters, my problems seemed miniscule after seeing what Jean had on her plate. Mother could at least hold a fairly intelligent conversation. Although she did confuse things, she could make you believe she understood what was being said. Harold couldn't. He talked in the past and at times was incoherent. Jean told him who I was and it didn't register. He rambled on about things we had done forty years ago as if he was trying to explain who I was to a complete stranger. This man had been the sheriff of a large county with a large staff for 12 years. Now, in just a very short time, he was reduced to almost a non-being. It broke my heart and made me cringe when I suddenly realized that I could have this in my future. Fortunately Mother never progressed to this state, but I had no way of knowing whether she would or wouldn't.

Harold's window had closed, and closed quickly. He was only 58 when his problem started and the disease took him in short order. He wandered and had to be restrained and closely watched. He lost motor control and had to be bathed, dressed, and helped with his toilet needs. He lost all recognition and didn't even know his wife at the end. The disease attacked his health and that hastened his demise.

The hardest part about caring for an Alzheimer's victim is the uncertainty of what is coming next. I was beginning to realize that every case is similar yet is in many ways...oh so different! If you, my reader, ever find yourself in the position of caregiver, expect the unexpected and it will always appear. All anyone can do is give you a pattern and most caregivers have a different pattern to give. Having said this, don't stop asking others for suggestions. I gleaned helpful advice every time I asked.

After leaving Harold's house that one time I never saw him again. Although he lived for several years, visiting him had stressed me and I decided visits did neither of us any good. In fact, it did me harm. I did keep up with the progress of his illness through neighbors and mutual friends and felt very lucky that Mother wasn't on the same fast downhill slide. I counted my blessings and continued my humble search for information that would aid me as I cared for Mother.

I read the book "The 36-Hour Day" and found it to be informative but clinical. I recommend it as "must" reading for anybody who becomes a caregiver. On a number of occasions during my four years of dealing with the three-minute window, I called the Helpline at the local chapter of the Alzheimer's Association. Every time the same thing happened. The caregiver I spoke with had never experienced the same problem that I was having, but we always had lengthy discussions. I usually came away with something else to expect. I also became aware of the fact that this disease had many faces. This makes it unpredictable and makes the caregiving job even harder. One day Mother would sit quietly gazing at the TV or looking out the window. The next day she would be in a nervous frenzy, trying to rearrange everything in the house.

My saving grace was the ever-present three-minute window. When frenzy set in, distraction was my tool. I would divert her attention to something in the yard or in a magazine or on television; usually she would forget what she was doing and settle down. She loved her back yard. Sometimes I would take her for a walk and pick a flower or two, then go back inside and arrange the flowers. She was a very artistic flower-arranger and could be counted on to explain to me that flowers should always be grouped in odd numbers...one, three, five and so on. And she would invariably tell me that my grandmother always said, "no flowers were better than dead flowers". As complicated as life might seem, it can usually be reduced to a simple handful of flowers if arranged in odd numbers and kept fresh. How do I know? My mother said so!

Chapter Four

Avoiding A Trip To Bonkersville!

If you become someone's caregiver, you must think of your well-being as much as the well-being of the person for whom you have assumed responsibility.

Before going any further, let me stress that every caregiver is an individual with a life of his own. If you get caught up in this situation, you must think of your well being as much as the well being of the person for whom you have assumed responsibility. You must find ways to isolate yourself from the situation from time to time or you will go completely bonkers! After a very short period of repetitive questions, confusing conversations, and unexpected situations, you start to question your own sanity. You have to find diversion and ways to occupy your mind or you'll be hauled off in a straight jacket. Here are a few ways I devised to maintain my mental health while still staying in control of the duties at hand.

When I was a young boy I started digging a basement under our house. It turned out to be just a big hole in the ground and was still just a big hole when I returned years later. I decided that the house needed a basement, so I set out to finish the job. It was a perfect diversion because it was good exercise, and since the house had wooden floors, I could hear Mother's every move. The tap...tap...tap of her cane was as good as radar or sonar to tell me which way she was headed. Of course I had to emerge frequently to check on her and make sure she wasn't into something that would either harm her or frustrate me.

My first job was to remove 40 years of tuck-away. Mother was a dyed-in-the-wool packrat. She had a rule that she lived by: if it wouldn't fit up the steps to the attic, stick it under the house! Ladders, old shingles, several decades of old automobile license plates (Virginia has two per car), junk that she had dragged from my uncle's hardware store, a stack of five-gallon buckets, and too much more stuff to mention had to be hauled out and disposed of or stored elsewhere. The buckets came in very handy because I used them to haul the dirt out as I dug. Every now and then she would wander onto the side porch next to where I was working and question what I was doing. Usually before I could answer she would return to her rocker with her question unanswered.

This project lasted a whole year because I used it to relieve tension and didn't turn it into a full-time job. My biggest problem was disposing of the dirt. The further down I went, the more the dirt turned into red clay. Red clay gets messy when it rains, so I had to find a way to cover it up. I built a low wall of concrete blocks behind the porch. That is where I built the stairs to the basement. This allowed me to fill in the area with the clay and eventually pour a concrete floor, turning it into a raised patio. I only dug a quarter basement because of the logistics. This project took more planning than physical work. It also became a fascination for the neighbors. Everybody wanted to see what I was doing and kept me company. Having a person nearby who could carry on a rational conversation was a blessed relief!

I mixed and poured all of the concrete by hand. The house was built on a raised brick foundation and was well supported. I allowed a foot between the foundation and where my "hole in the ground" was dug to avoid a cave-in. All I needed was a sunken house with Mother inside!

After the basement was complete, I built a small workshop in the basement where I could tinker. I had some electronic equipment and was given more, so I could escape downstairs and still listen to Mother's movements when I needed a bit of solitude.

Mother was a very frugal person who never owned a washer or dryer. She took great pride in never needing creature comforts. I always said that it was her burlap underwear. Anyway, I needed all the help that I could get. So my next door neighbor, Perry, came to my rescue. He knew someone who had a washer that was being discarded because it didn't work. He knew that I could fix things, so he arranged for me to get it. It served two purposes: a diversion, and if I got it fixed, a washer! I found that a very small screwdriver had become lodged in the pump and jammed the impeller. It had also caused a small puncture in the plastic wall of the pump. I removed the screwdriver, fixed the hole in the pump, and ZAM, I had a washer that was still working when Mother passed away three years later. I set it up in the new basement. Then, lo and behold, the same person who gave me the washer decided to get a new dryer and gave me the old one. Down in the basement it went, next to the washer.

Mother loved to hang clothes outside, but it took her forever with her condition. Every now and then we would hang a load out together. Then she would look out of the back window, see the clothes, and make a trip out to see if they were dry. During the course of one load drying, she would make a dozen of her slow, cane-assisted trips to the clothesline. It gave her something to do besides sit and rock, and I really think that the stimulation was good for her, although it caused me a little stress worrying about her hurting herself. When I saw her starting to take clothes off the line, I went out and helped. Usually the clothes were dry and ready to come in. But thank God for the dryer most of the time! After several years Mother's motor control got so bad that we had to stop this exercise.

Another diversion was the garden. Mother had been an avid gardener all her life and had a true green thumb. I have said many times that she could put a stick in the ground and it would sprout. I had never been much of a gardener, although I was brought up in a farm environment. Even though it wasn't my cup of tea, I figured it would be good for Mother to be able to pull a few weeds and pick a handful or two of fresh vegetables...if I could even get anything to sprout!

My oldest daughter, when visiting Mother as a little girl, said that she would hate to be a weed in Grandma's garden!

The first year I borrowed a tiller from my cousin. I had to do some work on it, but after getting it to run, I tilled a generic, straight-row garden. Luckily, I got corn, tomatoes, yellow and zucchini squash, butter beans, string beans, and beets to grow. I was a proud and happy camper! Mother already had a strawberry patch; it had been recycled so many years that the berries were very small. And she had a clump of asparagus that also came back each year. She really seemed to enjoy fiddling in HER garden. She thought that she had put the garden in. I let it be because there was no reason (or no way) to change her mind. I was amazed at my accomplishment. Working in the garden was another very therapeutic diversion. I decided that I had been missing something and started making plans for next year's garden.

Things always seem to fall into place, for some strange reason. I saw a picture in the newspaper of a friend I hadn't seen in many years. Jane used to visit Mother from time to time but hadn't seen her in several years. She was sitting on her tractor in the picture and the article was about her gardening accomplishments. So I decided to go visit Jane when I got the chance.

One day I got my neighbor Perry to keep an eye on Mother and I showed up on Jane's front porch. We had one very interesting commonality: my uncle married her aunt and we shared cousins. The cousin sharing was my introduction, but I still had to tell her who I was. This was the most important visit that I made during my entire caregiving days! You will hear the name, Jane, throughout this book because she became my main source of support and I can't give her enough thanks.

During the conversation I told Jane about my Mr. Fix-It gift and about my garden. She asked if I had a tiller. I told her I didn't but sure needed one. As luck would have it, she had an old tiller that had been sitting in the field for several years. She said that I was welcome to it but it probably wouldn't run. We went to the field, loaded the tiller in my van, and now I had another diversion!

I converted the tiller to an all-electronic ignition for a very small investment and in no time at all, I had a great little tiller. It was still running seven years later when I gave it to the person who bought our house. We moved into a community where I couldn't use it, but it served me well for years.

The next year's garden was more elaborate. I thought it would fascinate Mother. I combined flowers and vegetables in meandering, curving rows with wide walk spaces so she could navigate with her cane with no problem. She liked the flowers and the vegetables, but I don't think she ever realized that the layout was artistic. Oh well, I had fun doing it!

Jane got me involved in the County Master Gardeners course, which I needed desperately. With Perry watching our house after Mother had gone to bed (she tucked in early every evening), I would go once a week for two hours. I met a bunch of really nice people, got a break in the routine, and learned which end of the hoe to use. I never even came close to gaining Mother's gardening skills, but I learned enough to allow me to ask semi-intelligent questions when the need arose. Of course, when I returned to Florida most of my knowledge was lost on the different soil, different flora, and different climate. But I still have a certificate that tells the world that I am a Master Gardener, so I can hum a few bars and fake it.

Through my friendship with Jane, I got involved in composting, organic gardening, and raising Shiitake mushrooms. I developed a small, inexpensive composter and sold plans for others to build. All of this kept my mind active and kept me going when it seemed that I was trapped in an inescapable situation. Any activity that diverts your attention is like a gift from Heaven and is priceless.

I helped Jane do seminars on how to inoculate logs for Shiitake mushroom growth and how to cultivate and harvest them. I designed promotional and instructional material that she used for the seminars and learned quite a bit while doing it. When I could get Perry to keep an eye out for Mother, I would go to the woods and help cut logs. This was great exercise. Using the chain saw gave me a release for pent-up emotions, anxiety, and, yes....anger. Whether you want it to or not, anger creeps in because you are human. If you ever become a caregiver, get it out whenever you can. If nothing else, hang a rug up and beat it silly!

Jane sold Shiitakes to health food stores. I would leave home before daybreak while Mother was still asleep and harvest them for her. I also helped soak and stack the logs during the cultivation period. During the cultivation process you have to jog the logs on a hard object such as a concrete block to activate the seedlings. This was another energy release that reduced my stress. I would always be home way before Mother arose, but it was always on my mind so I hurried like crazy. Even when you are away, your caregiving duties are always foremost in your thoughts. This is stress you cannot avoid but will have to learn to handle.

When I first arrived to care for Mother, I had a very small-capacity computer and cheap printer. Needing some source of income, I set up an office in my bedroom and produced newsletters. After my friendship with Perry developed, we discovered a common interest in many things, especially computers. Although there was an age gap of 25 years, we established a bond that lasts to this day. He helped me upgrade to a larger computer and a better printer. We worked together to become very computer-literate. We connected our offices with an intercom and worked together on many projects. The computer became another diversion in which I could submerge myself, right in the house! Mother would peek in the door occasionally but never came in. All of this technical stuff in her house was confusing to her...so back to the rocker she went.

After a year had passed, along came Herman. Jane's beagle, Beulah, fell in love with a Labrador Retriever and produced a litter of five beautiful pups. Since the biggest one looked like a Herman to her, Jane named the boy dog that and insisted that he be mine. I have always been an animal lover, so I was very pleased to take him and watch him grow. And grow he did! In no time he turned into an eighty-pound giant and almost ate me out of house and home. He was great company and even Mother, no great dog lover, took to Herman. Since she never liked dogs in the house, Herman lived outside. I built a doghouse and a little fenced-in area where he grew up. When he got gigantic, he moved to a very long chain in the back yard and became friends with every kid in the neighborhood...and a lot of grown-ups also. His very presence was good for my state of mind. We would take walks together for great exercise and relaxation.

Neighbors, relatives and friends really helped to break up the monotony. Mother's backdoor neighbor, Beverly (who became my wife after Mother passed away) would come over and work puzzles with Mother. This gave me an opportunity to do things without having to worry about what was happening. Mother loved to work puzzles. Beverly found that she could find pieces and show Beverly where they went, but her motor skills had deteriorated and she couldn't insert the piece.

My cousin, Virginia, who lived several doors away, would stop by to visit two or three times a week. Having a third person in a conversation was very helpful and relieved some stress. It was good for my sanity to have somebody else hear the repetition and answer the same questions over and over. Other visitors were most welcome also.

These were my ways to stay sane. Since we are all so different, these things are only examples of what you can do. You need to provide a refuge to duck into when things start to bear down on you. In my case I was very lucky. Mother was not a roamer and, for the most part, was very docile. She stayed in the house and the yard and only got lost once in four years. Some victims are really a handful. The make their caregivers to be very creative to plan the occasional escape. Regardless of the situation, you must always remember that you are an individual and deserve a life of your own. Don't be a martyr. Call on anybody you can for help...family, neighbors, the church, support groups...anybody that can shield you occasionally from mental anguish. One day it will all be over and you can carry on. Be able to do just that!

Chapter Five

Please Don't Pull The Patch Off!

*This period was a terrific indoctrination
for what lay ahead during the years to come.
Every day brought a new challenge
to overcome.*

The reason I had come back to Virginia was to care for Mother after she had cataract operations. Of course, after I saw the situation, my job expanded from nursemaid to permanent caregiver. I never realized what a job my first mission would be! One of Mother's retinas turned out to be badly damaged early in life. This meant that she couldn't have the second eye operated on. She had worn glasses since she was in her twenties and no doctor had ever mentioned the damage before. It seems that during the many eye exams she had been through, someone should have discovered the problem. Her ophthalmologist said that the eye could have been corrected if it had been caught sooner. Not wishing Mother poor vision, but after what I went through with the first eye operation…all I could do was thank God for small favors!

Thinking back, I believe I might know when Mother's retina was damaged. The first year that our community had a church softball league, she went to a game at the high school I attended. She was standing behind third base. A batter swung at a pitch and the bat slipped out of his hands. It hit Mother on the bridge of her nose, breaking her glasses and driving the nosepiece into her nose. She had bone fragments picked from her nose several times in years to come. To show you why my mother was so loved and respected: a collection was taken at the next game to pay for her glasses and medical bills. A committee brought the collection to our house and was met at the door by Mother. She thanked them profusely, then handed the money back and told them to put up a fence at the ball field! I played sports on that field for a number of years and never saw that fence without thinking of my mother. Anyway, I think that blow in the face probably damaged the retina.

My Aunt Hazel took us into Richmond several times to see the ophthalmologist. I had been away for so long that I really had to learn the whole area again. I didn't feel comfortable handling Mother and finding a parking place on the busy streets. Mother couldn't remember that she had cataracts but was very good during the doctor's examinations. She continually complained about having a film over her eyes and would rub them trying to remove the film. I didn't realize at the time what a problem this was going to pose for me. The doctor had a very good "bedside manner" and was patient as Mother asked the same questions over and over.

Several years after Mother passed, I had to have cataracts removed from both of my eyes. I joked that I had caught my cataracts from Mother. As my eyes became cloudier and cloudier, my understanding of Mother's problem increased exponentially. The film that she kept complaining about became apparent; when she was experiencing it. I had no idea what she was talking about. Mine seemed more as though I were looking through a bottle of iodine. It would have been very helpful if I could have gone through this before Mother's ordeal. Being thrust into this completely foreign chore was very frustrating and made me wonder what I was in for in the future.

Finally the day came for the operation. Hazel took us to the hospital and waited with me during the surgery. Mother did well, and soon it was time to take her home. She was partially sedated and had no idea where she was or what had just happened to her. As the doctor had told us on every visit, she had a patch and eye shield on and it had to stay for ten days. My main job was to keep the patch and eye shield on Mother's eye. It was like trying to shave a wildcat in a phone booth with a dull razor!

When she first got home, we put her to bed and she slept off the sedation. It appeared to a naïve me that this was going to be a piece of cake. As soon as Mother awoke, I found out what a challenge I had ahead for me. She went into the operation with two eyes that allowed her partial vision. Now she had one bad eye and one covered, so she couldn't see at all. And she had no idea what had happened. All of the explaining in the world did no good because of her faulty memory. She started immediately to pull the patch off and I had my hands full from that moment on.

One saving grace was Mother's deep sleep patterns while she was on the pain medication. She slept soundly from the time she went to bed until she awoke, usually 12 hours later. During her sleep she didn't bother the patch. I had feared the worse but was spared. While she was awake, however, she was constantly fussing with the patch. I would help her get her glasses situated over the patch and shield, but she would forget and I had to watch her every moment. The first several days I would get her to lie on the couch so I could sit nearby and keep reminding her why the patch was there. She couldn't remember that she had cataracts or an operation, so she couldn't understand what had happened to her vision. Once she got so frustrated with my constant badgering that she told me to tie her hands! Of course I couldn't do that. I doubt if it would have done any good anyway.

After seven days we took her back to see the doctor. The operation had been very successful. He removed the patch but left the eye-shield on. It was made of metal and had a series of small holes in it. This was supposed to give adequate vision while protecting the eye. At the time I couldn't understand why Mother kept complaining about the shield over her eye. But after I had my first operation several years later, I fully understood. It was like looking through a colander and was very distracting. So Mother kept trying to remove it and my problems continued.

Because of her condition, the doctor allowed me to be in

the examining room while he was working with Mother. Sometimes the funniest things happened. Although she couldn't see well, she could see enough to realize that the doctor was a very tall man. She mentioned it to him and he made a comment that sparked a very funny statement from my mother. He said that he was tall, but he also had a long neck, which made him look even taller. Out of the blue Mother said, "Why don't you tie a knot in it?" We all had a good laugh and this was the doctor's conversational icebreaker on every visit after that.

A cataract operation like Mother's actually removes the old darkened lens and replaces it with a new man-made lens. The new lens is stitched in and has to heal completely before the stitches are removed. The doctor actually gave me the old lens and I kept it to show Mother when her vision returned. It looked like a small capsule filled with iodine. No wonder she could not see! The eye cannot be rubbed while the healing process is going on. Even if you have your full memory capabilities, it takes some restraint to keep from wanting to tamper with the eye. As it is healing, it itches. So I spent the longest two weeks of my life fearing every minute that the lens would be disturbed.

Another problem that Mother couldn't understand was that her glasses prescription had to be changed for the new lens. The eye shape changes during the healing process, so the glasses cannot be changed until the healing is complete. So she continually complained about fuzzy vision and couldn't remember what was going on. She didn't read much anymore, but she was always looking at magazines. I could tell that it made her very nervous that she had problems seeing. I really had to watch or she would remove the shield. The glasses fit tightly over the shield and she was constantly pulling off her glasses to wipe them with a Kleenex. I had the shield taped well, but she dragged the glasses, and on several occasions she actually ripped it off. I helped raise two children and never had a problem like this. I prayed for time to pass.

Mother had to return to the doctor quite a few times. Finally it was my turn to take her without Hazel's help. I drove a big van, and getting her into and out of the van was quite a task. She wasn't steady on her feet and she couldn't see that well, so I had to improvise. I got a big block of wood that would fit under the seat. On the ground it became a handy step. I would steady her as she went up the step to the van step and into the seat. Mother became very nervous when she had to travel, so I had this to contend with also. She would ask many times on the trip where we were going. Two minutes after I told her, she would forget and ask again. This, and the traffic, and finding parking on the street, and getting her in and out of the van made me very anxious to get back home!

On top of all of this, I had to deal with the insurance and make sure that the bills were paid. Mother had a Medicare supplement and the paperwork was so confusing that I wanted to scream. My bookkeeping skills were questionable; I really had to concentrate. We were living on such a tight budget that no mistakes could be tolerated. I learned that even large insurance companies were not infallible when I caught several errors that had to be corrected. The doctor's bookkeeper was a great help and I leaned on her to get through this dilemma.

The eye healed well and the time came for glasses to be fitted. Now that the shield was off, Mother was complaining that her glasses were blurred. This was because she basically had a new eye and an old prescription, but she couldn't remember that no matter how many times I told her. She cleaned and cleaned the glasses to no avail. I couldn't wait to get the new glasses.

It wasn't that easy. If you have ever had your eyes examined, you remember the "which is better...1 or 2?" tests. Well, Mother couldn't remember which was better! The doctor worked and worked and I have no idea how he succeeded in getting the new prescription correct. He clicked and clicked, moving from one setting to another. It frustrated him, exasperated Mother, and drove me up the wall! I know that I have trouble telling which setting is better, and I have my memory intact! After he got what he said were correct readings, we still had to wait about a week for the new glasses to be ready. So we were back to the blurred vision and the constant cleaning.

When we finally went back for the new glasses, I was amazed when the doctor slipped the glasses on Mother and asked her to read the chart. She could read a surprising amount of the smaller letters and we were told that this would get even better with time. My hat goes off to that fine doctor! As far as I was concerned, he had performed a miracle. Part of my nightmare was behind me now and I was very thankful. Now Mother could entertain herself to a certain extent by looking at her magazines and watching the world go by out the front window.

Because Mother still had a bad eye that could never be corrected, she still complained about having a film over her bad eye. She cleaned her glasses more than was necessary, but she could see. I had made it through my first assignment!

There was some good and some bad associated with her new vision. The good was that she amused herself by looking at things that she couldn't see before. The bad was that she began to get into things that she hadn't before. She moved around more and I never knew what she would do next. Some things she did didn't matter, but I never knew what to expect next. Bless her, she didn't mean to be a problem, but she could do some very strange things sometimes.

I had lived through the patch. This period was a terrific indoctrination for what lay ahead during the years to come. Every day brought a new challenge to overcome. Most of you will never experience something like my problem with Mother's eyes, but I'm here to tell you that you too will have a story to tell if you are (or become) a caregiver. Stay positive and you'll make it just fine!

Chapter Six

How Many More Stale Cheese Sandwiches Will I Find?

Every case has its own characteristics with some similarities, so there are no hard-and-fast guidelines. Caregivers have to play it by ear and develop their own guidelines.

Mother had been in a declining state of mind for a number of years when I arrived. She had squirreled away strange things. From time to time, she had simply forgotten what she was doing and left things in other than predictable places. After finding several items, I started searching as I tried to find where things I needed were kept so I could manage the household. Mother had always been a very orderly person, but now there was a degree of disorder because she couldn't remember where she kept things. A pattern developed that almost traced the downward spiral of Mother's memory.

One day I pulled the dining-room drapes over the radiator that heated the room. On top of the radiator cabinet lay a cheese sandwich, so stale that you couldn't cut it with a chain saw! No telling how long it had been there or why she had put it there. It seemed she hid things for future needs, evidently realizing that bad times were coming. So I started looking for other sandwiches. I found a total of ten! They were stuck in drawers, in cabinets, behind things on her sideboard, and even under her bed. They were always cheese. I know that Mother liked cheese as much as I do, and I think that some of them were laid down and just forgotten. She would become distracted and simply walk away. It is good that they were cheese and not meat! Can you imagine what a spoiled meat sandwich would have been like?

The next things I found were wads of chewing gum. Hard as a rock, they were neatly piled in the kitchen cabinet behind cans of food. They were also in the other cabinet behind the dishes. I don't know if she ever chewed them again. I certainly hope not! I remember when I was in grade school we used to stick chewing gum under the desk so the teacher wouldn't jump us for chewing in class. We just stuck it there and left it. Mother's gum wads were in neat little piles, the way squirrels pile their nuts. Here again, I have no idea how long they had been there. When I got there she had no gum and had a tooth that was loose so she refrained from chewing gum. She couldn't remember who had just visited, but she could remember not to chew gum. Go figure! Several years later the tooth fell out, but she never wanted gum again. Her doctor had told me just to let the tooth alone and it would come out by itself. It did...two years later.

It was evident that Mother realized her memory was waning. She left herself reminder notes. I found one that had all the names of the characters in one of her favorite soap operas. One had the mileage of the car she had given away five years before. In the last year she had put on a total of only 978 miles! It made her nervous to drive; the low mileage was evidence of that. Another note listed the names of all her relatives and who was whose child. She had notes about what service people did what kind of work. This was a smart thing to do, but she had stuck that note between her place mats in the sideboard drawer! She would have never found it if she had needed it.

That sideboard now sits in my living room. It brings back many memories; I can see it from the corner of my eye as I sit watching TV. In fact, now it is part of my entertainment center. It has been in the family since the 1820s and is probably the oldest electronic entertainment center in captivity today. I converted it without damaging any of its antique qualities. It has three door-concealed cabinets beneath two drawers. I made the center door so that it opens slowly when I press a switch beside my rocker. Then with a remote control I can tune an AM-FM stereo tuner, select one of three CDs or two cassettes, and control the volume and tone. Speakers propagate sound from beneath the sideboard and are located in each of the side cabinets. Even with its conversion, I still think of Mother's little notes all the time.

Mother and I became packrats naturally. My grandfather (her father) was a Scotsman and saved everything. As a boy, the highlight of my life was to get to go into his trunk with him. When you lifted the tray you saw a world of treasures. There were such valuable things as a cigar-shaped roll of tin foil saved from cigarette packs and gum wrappers. During the Second World War, this stuff was saved and sold for a small price to aid the war effort. Another marvelous thing was a gigantic ball of string. It was many short pieces tied together and wound into a ball. Granddaddy was a tobacco farmer and called the string 'bacco twine. It was used to tie leaves to the stick that was used in the curing process. It was all stained with tobacco wax and was totally useless...but it made a nice ball! We kids were always offered hard candy that had been in the trunk so long that it was all stuck together. We ate it anyway! Then there was a pouch full of pennies. We were paid in pennies for catching tobacco worms. Being a typical Scotsman, my grandfather's fee was one penny for 100 worms. It took forever to catch 100, but we did it anyway. And he actually dumped the worms out and counted them.

Mother and I joked about that trunk on many occasions. She could remember the past vividly and had loved that trunk too when she was a kid. We laughed often and said how much we loved that old man! He facetiously called his farm Mount Misery. And I have always referred to the trunk as "The First National Bank of Mount Misery"! He was my inspiration when I was growing up. I would kid Mother about her packrat habits and she would always say, "You never know when you're going to need something!" That has always been my philosophy too. We agreed and had another chuckle.

The next thing that I found was worth something. Mother had investments in CDs and got quarterly dividends. I came across one that was two years old. Printed right on the check it said "Must be cashed in 90 days". It was a nice sum of money and my heart sank. We could certainly use that money. I figured that I'd pursue it with the bank. I certainly couldn't lose more than was already lost. I took it to the bank and explained Mother's condition. She had been a customer for many years and the person with whom I talked was very understanding. She cashed the check for me. All Mother's accounts were in both of our names, so I could endorse the check. Needless to say, I went home and kept looking, hoping to find another check. Never did.

My first trip to the attic was a true revelation. Mother was a fireplace fanatic. She loved to build fires during the winter, so she collected kindling. When I was young, we went into the woods and got a small maple tree. It was planted in the back yard. After these many years, the trunk was about six feet in circumference and massive. It continuously dropped dead limbs into Mother's yard. Being a neat person, she couldn't stand a stick in her yard. So they went into grocery bags and, you guessed it...into the attic. There were 42 bags of sticks piled in the attic! When it came time to start a fire she would forget that the sticks were in the attic, so she would go out and get more sticks. Mother also disposed of her trash by using it as kindling. There was more than sticks in the attic, but that's a story within itself and will be covered in a later chapter. What a fire hazard! About ten years before, there had been a fire in the chimney. The fire department had to come and put the fire out. At that time they cautioned Mother about putting highly-flammable objects in the attic, but of course it had slipped her mind.

I had to sneak up there because she had been told by her doctor that, since she was on medication, she shouldn't go up the steps to the attic. It took me several days to tote all those bags outdoors. I created a dry place to store them and emptied the bags. Mother continued to bring in the sticks, but I persuaded her to put them in the wood tray by the fireplace. As the pile grew, I would move them out and she never knew the difference. You learn how to manage situations since the Alzheimer's victim can't remember from minute to minute. So you make the best of it.

Another strange thing that I found I have never figured out to this day. I don't know what possessed Mother to keep a lot of things, but this took the cake! Behind Daddy's picture on her dresser there was a container. I was straightening the things on her dresser and came upon it. Being nosey, I opened it. It was packed full of Mother's hair! When she brushed her hair she pulled the loose hair from the brush and stuck it in the container. Why I'll never know, unless she feared becoming bald and thought she'd need to have a wig made. I put the top back on and let it be. I figured that it couldn't hurt anything, so I left it. As time went on and her memory got worse, she finally stopped saving hair. And the mystery will never be solved. You can expect peculiar things like this and I guarantee that you will find plenty.

Mother was constantly rearranging things in her clothing drawers. Then she would get frustrated because she couldn't find things. I spent many hours helping her look for stuff that she had moved. She was constantly losing her pocketbook. Her pocketbook was her security blanket and she would simply come unglued when she couldn't find it. She would hide it in the closet, under the bed and under clothing in drawers. No sooner I would find it than she would hide it again. She kept saying that "they" were going to steal it. The game was never-ending! Her rearranging kept her busy and I felt that it was better for her to be doing busy work than to be just sitting and rocking. I never interfered and never criticized her for "losing" things. You can bet that it took a bunch of discipline to keep my cool, but I managed.

After Mother got used to my being there, she didn't write as many notes. The note-writing became my thing to do. You have probably read or heard that a big help in caregiving is to leave notes to help the victim know what to do. This is true. It really helps to post little reminders such as "Don't forget to brush" on the mirror in the bathroom or "This is for lunch" on a sandwich in the refrigerator. Some cases are so bad that this doesn't work. My friend, Harold, couldn't make sense of notes and couldn't be reasoned with, so he had to be led around and fenced out of certain areas. I was really lucky that Mother never got that bad. Every case has its own characteristics with some similarities, so there are no hard-and-fast guidelines. Caregivers have to play it by ear and develop their own guidelines.

It took me almost six months to find all of the stale cheese sandwiches, wads of chewing gum, balls of hair, bags of sticks, and other things that Mother had squirreled away. In fact, after Mother passed away and the house was being prepared for sale, things still popped up! Mother's condition spanned almost six years before I came onto the scene, so she had plenty of time to hide stuff and misplace things. This experience made me realize what a valuable asset a properly-functioning mind is. Everything really goes out of whack when you lose the ability to keep your thoughts straight and to recall things that you need to remember. Most people get a little forgetful as we get older, but there is a definite difference between forgetfulness and dementia. If you have any suspicions about anyone close to you, get a doctor's opinion. Alzheimer's disease is still not fully understood, so you won't get a definite diagnosis, but you will get a clue. Keep your eyes open and you will soon know whether you have something to worry about. I certainly hope that you never do!

Chapter Seven

I Wonder What's In The Attic... Besides Mother!

There are certain things that you must do, whether you want to or not. It comes with the territory.

Mother loved her attic. Since she was an avid scrounger and packrat, the attic contained a motherlode of questionable treasures. She had lived in the house for 48 years when I came back, and stuff was still up there that had been hauled up when we moved in. As she used to say, "You never know when you're going to need something!" Now her attic had become off limits because she was on medication that could affect her balance. You accessed it by a disappearing stairway and it was pretty steep. But the attic being off limits didn't stop my mother. She couldn't remember or understand why now she couldn't do what she had been doing for 48 years. She used to hang clothes in the attic in the winter. As I explained in the last chapter, she stored her sticks up there. And she just liked to go up and look for things that she really didn't need. So the attic became a problem. Later I'll tell what I had to do to solve the problem.

But first, let me fill you in on what treasures really are. I had to sneak up there to remove the sticks, and that was no small task. The stairway pulled down in the hall that led to Mother's bedroom and the bathroom, so she was coming and going all the time. I had to wait until she took a stroll in the backyard and garden to bring down the sticks. Then I had to go out the front door to get to the place where I was putting them. It took ten times as long to remove the bags of sticks as it should have. Once or twice she came in while I was in the attic and tried to climb up. I had to do some fast talking to get her back to her rocker. Then I had to wait for her next trip before I could carry on.

Mother was an avid gardener and canned much of the produce that she raised. She kept her empty jars in the attic. In addition to the standard Mason and Ball jars, she had mayonnaise and pickle jars and any other kind that had a lid that was suited for canning. Jars were stacked from floor to ceiling in one part of the attic. And my cousin Virginia would bring her wine when she went shopping for her. Mother had been a teetotaler for years because my father drank and caused quite a bit of pain in the family. But Mother forgot all that when her memory started to go. There was a bunch of wine bottles mixed in with the canning jars. Don't know what she planned to do with them...but you can bet she wasn't going to throw them away. After I came I discovered that she would have a glass of wine, forget that she had, and then have another! No wonder there were so many bottles in the attic! I put an end to that by rationing her to one small glass a day so that I wouldn't have a double problem on my hands. I checked with her doctor and he said that a small glass a day would probably be good for her. Anyway, he said, it wouldn't hurt her. My grandmother (her mother) was also a teetotaler until her last years, when she started taking whiskey as medicine. She called it a dram or toddy and had quite a few drams in a day. But, really, when you're in your eighties, whose business should it be how many drams you have?

Back to the attic. When the house was built, there was a square hole with a trap door to get into the attic. Several years later the disappearing stairway was installed. It was narrower than the hole. Mother and Daddy had put an old wicker rocker up there when we moved in and it was still there. When the house was sold and I cleared it out, I had to take the rockers off the chair to get it down. It's on my front porch now and serves very well for a chair over 100 years old!

Mother alternated her summer and winter clothes between the attic and her closet. She never got rid of clothes, so she had some very outdated styles hanging up there. Now she stayed in her nightgown and robe most of the time, so she didn't need a complete wardrobe for either summer or winter. I called my Aunt Hazel. We sorted through the clothing and gave quite a few very good dresses, coats, hats and other apparel to her church to be distributed to the needy.

When I was a Boy Scout, the attic was our patrol meeting place. All the Wolf Patrol flags and signs were still in place. All my boyhood toys and books were neatly stacked and my little desk still had all my valuable treasures in the drawers. Pictures of movie and sports stars, my paper route collection book, a tool to pump up footballs and basketballs...all in place. You never know when you'll need stuff like this! Hanging in a clothes bag were my old Air Force uniforms which Mother had tailored for me. They really brought back memories! I had lost sixty pounds after my initial issue and went from a thirty-six inch waist to thirty-two inches. When she took the pants in, the rear pockets almost touched. Because I hadn't dieted under doctor's orders, I couldn't get a new issue. So they wound up in the attic and I bought new Blues.

Daddy closed his store when WWII started. Anything worth saving went into the attic. All his ledgers and receipts were packed in boxes. I perused the ledgers and saw everybody in the county to whom Daddy had extended credit. It really brought back the past. I found it very interesting to see the prices for items people were buying back then.

When the store stuff went into the attic, so did canned goods. About two o'clock one morning in the middle of summer of the first year we lived there, explosions woke us up. Daddy yelled out that the Germans were bombing us! Then the smell permeated the house and we went up the ladder to the attic. Two cans of sauerkraut had exploded and covered the ceiling. It took several years for the odor to subside.

I guess that all these memories were Mother's fascination with the attic. Her trunk was up there. She had traveled to our county with that trunk to teach school. There were things in it that she had brought with her. My baby books and all the shower cards and things relating to my birth were in the trunk. The hospital receipt from where I was born was yellow but very readable. The total blew my mind...just $6.58! Times sure have changed. Also in the trunk were all of my report cards from school. My second-grade teacher had scratched "whispers too much" and had written "talks too much"! That flaw follows me to this day. But it was nice to see that I got good grades, for the most part. When I started playing sports there was a drop, but not enough to cause too much concern.

When I explored the attic, I had to trick Mother. I would get her situated in her rocker and turn on the TV. Then I would quietly pull the stairs down, go up, and pull the stairs behind me with a rope. She would usually stay put for awhile, so I could spend some time looking around and quietly moving and rearranging things before I went back down. Usually, since Mother had always been frugal, she would turn the TV off if she was leaving the living room. I could hear when it was turned off and would move fast! Even if she saw me coming down I could distract her with conversation until I got the stairs put back. Nobody who knows me has really understood what I was going through. It sounds so bizarre that most people would think I was exaggerating. But it all really happened.

The attic was under an "A" roof and only the middle was floored. It was partly insulated with old insulation. A lot of heat escaped through the ceiling and out through the roof. So I had two projects. I insulated and then put a scrap lumber floor over the open rafters. This was a real logistical challenge. I had to get the insulation up into the attic and had to scrounge plywood to floor with. But first, there was much junk that needed to be discarded. I did this with a five-gallon bucket and a rope through the attic window. This was time-consuming, but I wasn't going anyplace. Stuff included several shingle sample displays, other display parts from my uncle's store, and an old burned-out barbecue grill that should have been tossed years ago... but remember Mother's motto! Of course, the wine bottles needed to go also. Perry, my neighbor, and I had bought a trailer that I used to haul the clutter to the county dump.

After I disposed of much stuff, there was still much stuff left. I had to move things from over the exposed rafters onto the floor so I could insulate and lay the floor. Mother was relentless in her efforts to go up into the attic. Several times I would come in and find her up there surveying the mess. She kept saying that she must straighten up the attic so she could find things. I would have to go through a routine to lure her back down and distract her so that she would forget the attic. I just knew that one time she would slip and fall, leaving me with a real problem.

I finally got the insulation down and the scrap-lumber flooring in place. I would go out early in the morning before sunup and get plywood from shipping boxes that was being discarded in dumpsters behind stores. One appliance store was a very good source. It seemed to take forever because I couldn't find large amounts, and I also had to pull nails and disassemble some box lids before I could use them. But I did get the partial floor down and moved most of the things back out of the walkway. Mother was still going up the stairs whenever I wasn't looking, so I hurried as much as I could.

After the bulk of the job was done, I decided that I would have to put a stop to the visits to the attic before Mother fell and caused a catastrophe. I screwed the pull-down stairway door shut so that it couldn't be opened. Of course I had to remove the screws every time I needed to go up. But it did stop her frequent visits. I watched several times and she would pull the chain, look puzzled when it wouldn't open, try again, then give up and move on to do something else. She never mentioned it to me because by the time I made myself available, it had slipped her mind. I really would like to have been able to penetrate her mind to see what she was thinking. She had always been a problem solver but now she was stymied. Not like my mother at all.

One time she really tried to get the door open. She actually pulled the chain so hard that it broke where it was attached to the door. I found the chain hanging on the knob on her bedroom door. I put it away and never put it back up. Without the dangling chain, the attic was out of mind, so I had eliminated another frustration. It made me feel badly that another one of Mother's favorite places was off limits, but it simply had to be. If you are a caregiver or become one, you will better understand the dilemma in which I found myself. There are certain things that you must do, whether you want to or not. It comes with the territory. I assure you that the person for whom you are caring has lost reasoning power and will only be put out for the moment. It is exactly like caring for a very young child, except that the child learns from the action. The Alzheimer's victim doesn't learn. Sad, but true.

Chapter Eight

Come Help Me Burn The House Down!

You never know what will happen next, so a caregiver has to be alert to everything.

When I got to Virginia, the weather was still on the cold side. I had become a typical Floridian and couldn't stand to be cold. The heat had to be on all the time and a fire in the fireplace was not only cozy and pleasant to look at, it helped keep you warm. Mother had always used the fireplace, even though she had almost burned the house down with it several years ago. She had to have the chimney rebuilt and a mechanical damper was installed at that time. It stopped the heat from the radiators from escaping when the fireplace was not in use. This hadn't been there when I was a boy living at home, so I wasn't used to it. It turned out to be the source of a near-disaster.

One day I suggested using the fireplace. Mother thought that would be really nice and told me about the damper. I don't know what reminded her, but in the early days of her problem, some things did remain in memory. Well, I removed the fire screen and a wooden cover that further preserved the house heat. I opened the damper and rounded up some kindling and wood for the fire. (At that time I didn't know about the 42 bags of sticks in the attic.) After I finished, I went into the kitchen for matches. Unbeknownst to me, Mother closed the damper. When I came back and started the fire...panic set in! Flames leaped out, licking at the mantelpiece. The paint caught fire and I was scared to death. I yelled at Mother to get some water. I took my shirt off and beat at the flames. Mother moved faster than I've ever seen her move! Several years later this wouldn't have been the case. Even with her vision problem, she was able to bring me a big kettle of water. The hot firescreen fell against my sweatpants and left a lasting imprint. If it hadn't been for the pants, I would have had a permanent scar.

The water saved the day. Mother returned to the kitchen for a second kettle and I got the fire out. The mantel was a mess and we had no fire. But I was satisfied not to have a cozy fire that day and closed the fireplace up. Mother was a nervous wreck. It took me awhile to get her settled down. This was, so to speak, my baptism of fire! You never know what will happen next, so a caregiver has to be alert to everything. After this, I checked and double-checked anything that could cause a problem. But I still ran into some situations that had potential catastrophe written all over them. Later we did use the fireplace quite often, but that damper was etched in my mind and a match was never struck until I made sure that it was open.

I had to remove the burned paint from the mantel and repaint it. What a mess! I had to scrape, sand, and sand some more. There was fancy trim molding with curves and grooves and many layers of paint. No telling how many times it had been painted over the years. I hate to paint, so that didn't make the task any easier.

The heat and smoke had also wrecked the brass andirons. Mother had an abundance of brass things that she used to keep bright and shiny. She had neglected them the last several years and they really needed attention. While I was cleaning the andirons I discovered that a little muriatic acid in water helped remove the oxidation easily. (If you try this, please be careful, because the fumes are toxic and the acid will burn you. Rubber or latex gloves are a must!) While I was into brass cleanup, I decided to clean all of the brass. Mother really liked seeing her candlesticks and pots and andirons shine again. That made the effort worthwhile.

A pretty gold-leaf framed mirror hung above the mantel and it was smoke-damaged, so I redid the frame also. Mother had waxed and re-waxed the bricks in the hearth many times over the years and the fire scorched the bricks. I removed every brick, turned them over, and redid the mortar. Mother seemed to enjoy watching me work. She sat in her rocker and commented many times how nice the mantel looked after I repainted it. She couldn't see it well, but she knew that it had been improved. She kept asking what had happened to the mantel. It was a sign of the future: questions, questions, questions! The same ones over and over.

After Mother's vision was repaired, I caught her several times at the fireplace with a full trashcan, burning the trash. For years this had been her method of trash disposal, both summer and winter. Matches were in the kitchen on the stove so she could get them easily. When I discovered what was happening I tried to keep the trash emptied, but sometimes I'd forget and the lady would be back at the fireplace. It became apparent that matches would have to be hidden if I wanted to keep the house intact. My room was the best place, because Mother would only come to the door and speak to me. She stayed out because of my computer and things that she would have nothing to do with.

Matches had been a part of Mother's life because she had cooked with gas, had a fireplace, and used candles as an accent to her interior décor. She wanted her matches and could not understand why she could never find one. My job was to make sure she didn't find them. Out of the blue she'd say, "We need to buy some matches. I've let them run out and I need one." It did no good to try and explain, so I'd simply nod my head and go on about my business. No one will ever know how much it hurt to have to treat someone that I'd respected all my life like that. Until her last days she would look for matches. Such a simple pleasure to be denied.

I finally installed a nice fire screen with tempered glass doors on the fireplace. This was mechanical in nature and Mother had started to shy away from anything mechanical. I can only surmise that it was because her motor skills had deteriorated and it made her nervous to work with things like the fireplace doors. The screen served two purposes. It made the fireplace look nice and it kept Mother out. She enjoyed watching a fire in the winter, but she left the tending up to me. I will never know why she hadn't accidentally burned the house down before I came to care for her. I guess the Almighty has a way of knowing who needs looking after.

The kitchen was another problem area. Mother still thought that she was the cook of the house. Truth is, her credentials sure overshadowed mine. But her thought process left a lot to be desired. Until I put a stop to it, she would put a pan of water on the gas stove, light it with the pilot light, and head for the rocker. You can bet that I found a few pans in pretty bad condition. She would take frozen things from the freezer, put them on the counter to thaw, and forget what was going on. This must have happened before I came back home and I don't know how she made out. Very dangerous situation indeed!

My first move to control the problem was totally stupid, now that I reflect on what I did. I shut the pilot off and had all matches out of sight. Mother simply operated by rote, since she had used that stove for many years. One day I came from outside just in time. There was a very strong gas smell in the kitchen. Mother was in her rocker and was out of range of the gas for the time being. I'm so glad that I came in when I did. She had turned the burner on expecting it to light as it always had, and left the kitchen. That really shook me up! Needless to say, I had to make other arrangements. I had to open the windows and doors to clear the gas from the house.

This was my first inconvenience. There would be more, but I had no choice. I had to disconnect the stove and cap the line because the water heater was gas also. At the time I had no microwave, just a toaster oven. When my neighbor, Perry, found out about the problem, he found a microwave that didn't work. He knew that I could probably fix it and I did…with a $2.80 part! It wasn't the same as having a range and oven, but I really didn't do much cooking. I did a lot of heating things up and the microwave and toaster oven served me well. Eventually I got an electric water heater and put it in the basement. It seemed to me to be more reasonable, cost-wise, than the gas heater. Mother had always used gas because she thought that she was saving money. I really wonder how much she had actually saved.

Although the toaster oven was Mother's, she never bothered with it. And the microwave was in the same category as my computer and other electronic stuff, so she left it alone too. I left the stove in the kitchen and occasionally found a pot of water on a burner with the control turned on, but now no damage could be done. I don't know how other caregivers handle this type of problem, since most people would not do without a kitchen stove. I'm sure that many women with Alzheimer's Disease have cooked all their lives. They must do things like Mother did and probably cause the same potential harm. Some caregivers simply shut off the kitchen. Any way you look at it, there is considerable inconvenience.

Another thing that never entered my mind was that Mother would try to get matches from visitors. After she realized whom she was visiting with, she could hold a conversation that was very convincing. Even in the later years, she could fool people that didn't know her well. A relative told me about the match episode. She said Mother had a story that could con most anybody out of a book of matches. It actually happened once and I found the matches on her dresser. Nothing was burned, but now I had to keep my eyes and ears open that much more. I tried to be with her when people came to visit, but sometimes that was impossible. I'm sure that many people thought I was the one whose mind had gone. Mother had always been a terrifically engaging conversationalist and never lost the talent. She never got that foggy look that so many victims develop. Because she appeared to be paying attention, you wouldn't know otherwise until she asked the same question several times. (Some perfectly healthy people I know do the same thing, but that's because they never pay attention!)

I used the fireplace and mantel story to make my point and try to convey a message when people came to see us. The interesting thing is that I could tell stories about things like that and Mother would listen, just as though she had never heard the story before...much less been a central player. Sometimes she would actually ask questions, as if she had been on another planet when the fire occurred. This made it even harder to convince other people that the story was true. Looking back on those years makes me wonder how I made it. Many of the things you are reading in this book have been conveniently buried in my subconscious mind to protect my sanity. There was a great amount of hurt involved. I'm having to dredge it up in hopes that some caregiver somewhere will benefit from my experiences. It is also giving me a degree of final closure that I had denied myself.

The only advice that I can give is to stay aware of everything. Note changes in any patterns that develop. Just remember that patterns related to this disease change like the wind and the shifting sand. Be open with everybody you come in contact with, so that people know your situation. Don't be embarrassed about the hand that has been dealt you or about what the victim says or does. Forgive them, for they know not what they do!

Chapter Nine

Doctor, Doctor...
Please Spare Me The Pain

I would like to point out that the caregiver's health is as important as the health of the one being attended. I can speak from experience.

Mother had a few cardiovascular problems that were being treated when I arrived. The cardiologist she was visiting was the one who had given the second opinion about her condition. He had said it was not necessary to do the recommended invasive procedure to break up the plaque in her carotid artery on the right side. This would have meant entering an incision in her groin and sending a device up to the problem area. A fifty-fifty chance existed that this could have been fatal. He won my approval; I maintained that at her age she didn't need to go through a painful operation that could end her life. So we switched cardiologists. For every plus there seems to be a minus, and after several visits I discovered the minus.

It turned out that closely-spaced visits were getting closer and closer. At first I could see the benefit of regular check-ups, because Mother's cholesterol was very high and she complained occasionally about a pain in her neck. The neck pain was where she had partial blockage of the carotid artery leading to the brain. We had been told that if we could control the cholesterol, the plaque build-up would not increase and the stroke danger would decrease. On each visit an EKG was performed and blood work was done. Mother was on medication to help the problem and it seemed to be working.

There seemed to be a bit of Medicare-milking going on. It didn't take me long to figure out what was happening. Every visit spawned another visit, or a trip to a lab or two for more tests. Mother was on medication that required doctor's approval for prescription renewal; that meant continuing visits. It seemed every time I turned around we were off to see the doctor. Of course, every visit meant a co-payment from us, and a payment to the doctor from Mother's Medicare supplement insurance company. I started to wonder if all these visits and tests were really necessary. Through diet, I had gotten her cholesterol under control and had her at an acceptable weight. Her hypertension was being controlled by medication and she seemed to feel very good. Her health was satisfactory for a person her age. But the visits continued.

I didn't want to do anything that would hurt Mother's health. My main problem was the total frustration of getting her to and from the doctor's office. It upset her so much when she had to get ready for the trip that I had to come up with a plan that would eliminate the pain for both of us.

She had developed urinary incontinence and it was embarrassing for her. This is a symptom of Alzheimer's Disease as well as being a function of old age. She wore old-fashioned diapers and would have nothing to do with the newer disposables, as advertised by June Allyson on TV. In fact, my cousin Carolyn bought several packages early in my stay and they were still in the cabinet when the house was cleared out for sale. Mother had always been militant against anything she considered too expensive or frivolous. She never changed! She had a rack in the bathroom and washed her diapers as she used them. I let her do this to keep her active, but she didn't do the greatest job so I had about three washdays a week.

As with all doctors' visits, the cardiologist was never on time for the scheduled appointment. Mother would get uncomfortable and annoyed. She would start fidgeting and complaining and that embarrassed me. I tried to distract her, but when you're sitting in a damp diaper, distraction is next to impossible.

I mentioned the problem to the doctor. I wondered if there wasn't some way to lessen the visits. He said that it was critical that Mother be frequently tested and monitored. I hate to be harsh on the medical community; I do appreciate what had been done to help my mother enjoy better health. But the fact is medicine is a business and the bottom line is extremely important. This is not true of all practitioners, but some ruin it for all.

My Uncle Luther was a doctor until he was 86 years old and he never put the dollar first. He was never wealthy but he slept well every night. And he was the only doctor with whom I have ever really felt comfortable. He was a simple talker and a straight shooter and he instilled an unshakable trust. The cardiologist's answer verified my conclusion that insurance checks were at the root of the frequent visits. I decided to find a better method of keeping Mother healthy.

The cardiologist was an Iraqi native. He was born and raised in Baghdad and was a graduate of Baghdad University. We had an appointment on January 16, 1991, the day the Persian Gulf War started. Ironically, Mother had one of her infrequent head colds and I wasn't about to take her out in the chilly weather. The news was blaring on TV about our bombing Iraq, and especially Baghdad. I called and cancelled the appointment and didn't make another. It didn't occur to me until later, but I'll bet to this day that the doctor thought I cancelled because of his ethnic background! We went back several times after that and his attitude was a bit different. Maybe it's my imagination, but I found him to be a little more sympathetic to my concern about the frequent visits. He cut back and let the pharmacy call for refills on her medicine. Amazing what can be done when you try a little!

At first, while we were making trips to the cardiologist, we were also visiting the ophthalmologist for the cataract problem. It seemed that every time I turned around we were loading up and heading to doctors' offices. For two people who really didn't like to see physicians, we were setting some kind of record. We continued going to the cardiologist well after the cataract episode was over. Mother took longer and longer to get her nerves unfrayed and my nerves were beginning to come unglued, too. At first, I started the day before trying to prepare her for the next day's trip. She would become visibly unraveled. As you know by now, in a short time she had forgotten, so it was a futile effort on my part. Then I would wait until she had just enough time to get dressed before I mentioned it. This upset her; she became confused and couldn't find things to wear. I tried to help, but a son has no place in his mother's bedroom as she is getting dressed, so I wasn't much help. By the time we were ready to leave, we were both in such a lather we weren't fit to go anywhere.

All these trips to the doctor took another toll that I wish could have been avoided. The family liked to have us to dinner and for special events such as birthdays, Christmas and the like. These events were enjoyable to me and Mother had always been socially inclined and fun for the family. Not only did I enjoy the company and good food, but also the family helped break my stress. During the first year we attended quite a few of these soirées and Mother handled them quite nicely. I had a little carrying-case for her extra toiletry needs, so she stayed comfortable. She was embarrassed by her problem, but she was with family and the ladies helped her in her times of need. Several times when I first got back, my cousin Carolyn would come and show us around Richmond. I knew little about changes that had taken place over the years, so it was really enjoyable. But the more doctor's office trips we made, the more reluctance Mother showed to travelling anywhere. In fact, in the beginning, Mother dressed every day, even if she was just going to stay in the house in her rocker. As time went on, she started to stay in her gown and robe more and more. Selfishly, it was easier on me, since I didn't have as many clothes to wash. But it really wasn't good for her, because dressing gave her a little challenge that she needed to stimulate her brain. So I would talk her into dressing several times a week, until she finally rebelled. I tried to take her for rides around the county, thinking that she would enjoy getting out occasionally. But when you can't remember what you just saw, there can't be much joy in Mudville! Would you believe that the medical profession could have caused these problems? Of course it wasn't intentional, but it sure did put more on my plate than I needed to deal with.

It tended to upset the family when Mother refused their invitations. I worried that they blamed me. It is hard for others to understand things like this. After two years, Mother got in such a tizzy every time a trip of any kind was mentioned I just gave up. Fortunately, people kept coming to see us, because Mother refused to budge. The only travelling she wanted to do was to take her slow-moving strolls into the back yard and the garden.

Her EKGs were greatly improved and her cholesterol count was low. Complaints of neck pain had stopped completely. She still had hypertension, but it was under control by medication. Since travelling had become such a problem, I had to find some way to keep getting her prescriptions filled. My friend Jane came to my rescue. She suggested that I call a local doctor who was a member of her church and the church where I had been an active member as a youth. Who says that doctors don't do house calls anymore? He got her records transferred, came to the house and gave Mother a very thorough examination and said that she was fit as a fiddle for her age. He told me what to look for, and to call him if any symptom arose and he would come back to the house. I breathed a sigh of relief. His office took care of the insurance forms and our travelling pain was gone! I felt that as long as I paid attention to her complaints, she was as safe as anybody could be. I thanked God in my simple way for people like Jane and Mother's new house-calling doctor.

After the initial diagnosis of early-stage Alzheimer's disease, I never bothered a doctor with this problem. Basically, I was told that there was no cure and that medical science knew little about the disease. The doctor said that if Mother sat and rocked and looked out the window, she was an Alzheimer's sufferer. And the more she sat and rocked and looked out the window, the worse the case was getting. Why spend money on a doctor when I could keep an eye on the rocking? In Mothers case, the rocking did increase as the years passed, but her health didn't deteriorate as badly as it does in many cases. Today medical science has more knowledge about symptoms and are working on possible cures. There is still plenty of mystery involved, but at least strides are being made to arrest this frightening illness and eventual killer. Caregivers should read as much as is available and check with a physician to see if anything can be prescribed to slow the progress of the disease. I just hope that you don't suffer the pain that I did when it came to going to the doctor.

I would like to point out that the caregiver's health is as important as the health of the one being attended. I can speak from experience. In my third year I developed a headache so severe that I had trouble seeing. Taking care of Mother was a real chore. On the twelfth day with no relief, I went to a chiropractor recommended by Jane. After much twisting, jerking and cracking, he told me that he feared a brain tumor. He made arrangements for me to go to the local Veterans Hospital for a CatScan. It turned out to be acute sinusitis and was cured quickly. Caregiving became much easier again and flagged me to stay healthy. "Doctor" took on new meaning for me!

Chapter Ten

A Very Puzzling Thing

Mother couldn't remember who had visited
or what she had eaten, but she could remember words
and their meanings with no problem. It amazed me!

Mother was an ardent puzzle-worker. She loved jigsaw and crossword puzzles and spent hours amusing herself most of her life. She was very good at it and was fascinated by words and word origins. I guess I inherited it from her, because I share that same fascination. After she was afflicted with Alzheimer's disease her motor functions started to fail her, but she could still find puzzle pieces and fit words with meanings in crosswords. In fact, she would work the same crossword puzzles over and over by just finding words and not filling them in. She had books of puzzles that my children had given her over the years. These books had the solutions in the back. She would figure out a word and write it on a piece of paper. Then she would check the answer. She did that so many times that the books were worn and dog-eared. She couldn't remember who had visited or what she had eaten, but she could remember words and their meanings with no problem. It amazed me!

The Richmond newspaper had a word puzzle called Jumbles. Mother enjoyed them and they kept her busy almost every day. She couldn't remember that she had worked the Jumbles, so I started making several copies of each one and she thought she had fresh ones all the time. She would ask me to help her with a certain word and would come up with the answer before I could even get my brain in gear! As the years passed, her word recall slowed considerably, but she could still find the word to fit the question. She would try to read an article in the paper and couldn't keep up with what she was reading, but when she worked one word at a time she had no problem. It was very baffling.

When I first came back to live in Virginia, I was trying to sell a newsletter by direct mail. I did mailings to purchased mailing lists. Usually there were three pieces that went into an envelope; then a label had to be affixed to the envelope. Mother saw me stuffing envelopes and said that she would like to help. It was a simple routine so I figured that she would have no problem. I set up a card table in front of her rocker and put the pieces in separate stacks.

There were two hundred mailing pieces in her project. I would go in at close intervals to check progress; she would be sitting and staring at the stacks. She would do two or three and forget what she was doing. Finally she got finished after many of my checking trips. I checked a few envelopes and they had two identical letters and a return envelope but no order form, or a letter and order form but no return envelope. I had to redo the whole stack and found out that Mother couldn't do even the simplest manual task. I guess it was a motor control problem. From then on I did my own envelope stuffing. According to the Clinical Practice Guideline, "Recognition and Initial Assessment of Alzheimer's Disease and Related Dementias," published by the U.S. Department of Health and Human Services, one of the symptoms is difficulty in following a complex train of thought or performing tasks that require many steps. Examples given are balancing a checkbook or cooking a meal. Mother hadn't done either in years.

Neither had she worked jigsaw puzzles by herself in quite some time. She couldn't put the pieces in place and for some reason couldn't find the outside pieces. On a number of occasions when I needed to go into the attic for an extended time, or had to do other things and needed a distraction for Mother, Beverly (my bride after Mother passed) would bring puzzles and work them with her. She had six small puzzles that Mother liked. She would put the outside together and Mother would find pieces and show Beverly where they went. It was spooky how often she was correct. She couldn't place the piece, or she had great difficulty doing it, but it was uncanny how she could match shapes. Beverly called the motor function to my attention. She was a Special Education teacher and had experience with that deficiency in children she had taught. It seemed that some of Mother's functions worked just fine, while others left a lot to be desired. I suspect that artistic ability helped her with shapes and especially with colors.

Mother had always enjoyed games that challenged her. Probably nobody reading this book has ever heard of a card game named "Logomachy", or "War of Words". It was created by the Milton Bradley Company and was the forerunner of Scrabble. I still have the game and it is ancient. It belonged to my father's mother and maybe her mother before that. Mother and I played it many times when I was growing up and she was an excellent player. One day I asked her if she'd like to play. Her eyes lit up and she smiled. So we did...or we tried. You built words off other words by laying the cards down to spell them. Mother could see the words in her hand but had great difficulty getting them lined up. She would get terribly frustrated, to the point of irritation. I finally gave that up as a bad idea. Her only times of aggravation were when she couldn't perform things that she had done so easily all of her life. I still choke up when I think about how this self-sufficient, talented woman became a shipwreck in her own body.

When the eye-to-hand coordination goes, a whole lot goes with it. Mother had problems buttoning her robe, although it had big buttons. She couldn't button a blouse whenever I could get her into one. She had threaded more needles in her time than you can imagine, yet now it was an impossible chore. She even had one of those needle-threading devices, but couldn't put that into the eye of the needle. She could arrange large things if there was no set pattern, like the maple leaves on the kitchen table. And she insisted on making her own bed every morning. It took her forever, but she did a commendable job. I am convinced that the reason that no more is known about this disease is because there is no rhyme or reason to it. Nothing is predictable. I hope someday mankind stops it in its tracks, but it may not happen in my lifetime.

Chapter Eleven

Tell Me That Story Again, Mother... And Again...And Again...

*Even when Mother's stories would get confused,
she still told them as if she knew
that every word was correct. If I corrected her,
she would become frustrated. It really didn't make
one bit of difference, I knew every story by heart
and she was enjoying telling her new version.*

A natural trait of older people is to dwell on the past. Short-term memory of the Alzheimer's victim gets shorter and shorter, while the past remains intact...for a while. Mother told the same stories over and over and as time went on, the stories became confused. She would misplace people and places. If I hadn't heard the stories since I was a child, I wouldn't have known the difference. I have always been fascinated by family tales and collected them in my mind over the years. Mother, too, was a good storyteller, so she had a storehouse of things to dwell on. You can bet that she did! After a while I thought, "If I hear that story one more time, I will scream!" I didn't, but I don't know how I controlled myself.

She would always say, " I can't remember...have I told you about so-and-so before?" Before I could say yes, the tale would start to spin. In 1923 she caught a train from her home in

South Hill, Virginia, and came to Richmond, where she took a bus to Old Church for a teaching job. We made that trip so many times during my caregiving days that I know every turn by heart! The road she took runs through the little hometown where she lived and is now a very busy highway. Back then it was a dirt road.

At the corner of the crossroads that led to where she would stay was a landmark known as "John West's Store". The old store is gone now, but a new West's Store replaced it and belongs to the same family. The lady with whom Mother was to board had hired a young local man to go to the store and pick her up. That young man was later to become my father. The punch line to Mother's story always was, "I met my Waterloo at John West's Store!" She really got a kick out of telling the story and always got a healthy chuckle out of it. That is one story that never got confused; it was probably the one event that would drastically change her life forever. I enjoyed it, I guess, because if it hadn't happened I wouldn't be telling you about it now.

As a caregiver, you have to be able either to tune out the stories or to be a good listener. I really think that as long as Mother told her stories, her dementia didn't get worse. I'm just guessing, because I don't think any scientific data support my belief. Anyway, when she had a day when she was a little more out of it than others, I would bait her. I would say, "Mother, remember when…" and she would start into a narration. Or I would get an item that had a story attached to it and ask if she knew where it came from or who gave it to her. I now have antique plates hanging on either side of her old sideboard that always triggered the same response back then. For some reason she could not remember where they came from, although she could tell you who gave her every other trinket that she owned. But she had evidently made up a story to fit the plates. She would say that someone brought her the plates and asked her to keep them until they came back. According to Mother, the person never came back. I asked family and friends, to no avail, if anybody knew where the plates came from. Suits me that nobody ever claimed them, but I sure would like to know the rest of the story.

Sometimes I thought she made up other stories, but I didn't question her, just let her tell the story. When I was ready to start school, the State of Virginia had a rule that you had to be seven years old for a given period of time before the school year started, or else you had to wait until the next year. My birthday was in April, so I wouldn't be seven until then and would have to wait the year out before starting. Mother thought that I was old enough to start, so she found a way around the rule. She had one of her old teacher buddies who was on maternity leave with her first child tutor me. When I reached seven, she had me "transferred" into the first grade. Slick trick! Well, Mother kept telling me that Ruby (my tutor) had come to see her not long ago. Her time reference was locked in place, so it seemed to her that it had been just yesterday. She said that a black lady had brought Ruby and that the lady sat in a particular chair (which she always pointed to) while Mother and Ruby visited. I really questioned the story until one day I actually got to visit Ruby. The first words out of her mouth after the normal salutations were, "I went to visit Cile several years ago. My nurse took me." All of Mother's friends called her Cile. The story was obviously true! From then on, when she told the story, which was quite often, she was telling a believer.

Another thing that seemed to stick in her mind were her pupils that she had taught many years ago. She didn't teach long, because back then Virginia law wouldn't let a married woman teach. She had to resign after she "met her Waterloo!" But she kept telling little vignettes of things her students had done and could name every pupil. All of them whom I have ever met thought the world of Miss Lucile and went out of their way to speak to her or do things for her. One of the students grew up to be one of the better farmers in our county. We had wonderfully sweet cantaloupes every summer as I was growing up. Several years ago, one of my cousins married his daughter, so now I guess we're all family. Mother would certainly approve, because she thought the world of Cary. As time passed, she would get the names confused with other people in her past, but she still loved to relive those old school-teaching days.

My mother and father had a very rocky marriage. It was never what you could call happy. They disagreed on everything and were fussing about something most of the time. Daddy drank, which displeased Mother to the point of tears. He was not a good money manager and there was constant friction about that. They started out their married life living with Daddy's mother and father and lived there for the first nine years. Daddy was Grandmother's pet. She caused many problems in the marriage by siding with her son and not letting them work things out for themselves. All in all, their marriage was a disaster. But Alzheimer's fixed all that. Mother would tell me time and again what a wonderful man she had married and how happy they had been. This was a part of the past that she never got right. I know, because I lived through it! When I would call her attention to certain things that had happened, she would say, "I wonder where I've been all of these years." I don't know whether it was a defense mechanism that she had built or what.

It was the same with Daddy's death. She found him that morning, but could not recall anything about the whole incident. I would say that maybe shock had done it, but for years before her dementia problem, she could tell you everything that had happened, right down to what the doctor had said about his massive coronary. There is no rhyme or reason to this disease and what it does to the mind.

Mother's favorite story was one her mother used to tell on her father. Grandma always claimed that Granddaddy was the laziest man on Earth and would do anything to avoid work. He had beehives and harvested the honey from time to time. On one occasion, he had been complaining about what he called "back misery". He was moping around and mostly sitting on his swing. She told him a hive needed tending. After much ado, he agreed that if somebody would set the hive on the front sidewalk and bring him a chair, he would take the honey. Grandma would start laughing at this point and could hardly finish the story.

Granddaddy wore bib overalls. Most farmers of that day wore them. It seems that he dropped a clump of bees inside the bib of his overalls. She said that he started circling the house taking off a layer of clothing on each pass. By the time he headed into the house, he was completely bare and moving at a very fast pace! She said that from that day forward she never heard another word about back misery. Mother loved to tell the story and we both always laughed throughout it. In my opinion, this was therapy that no medicine could replace. It always amazed me that Mother could maintain a train of thought when telling a story, even though three minutes later she had forgotten that a story had been told.

This little tale was always followed by Granddaddy's retort. Grandma's first name was Mamie, but he always called her "Miss Manie". When she finished her story and the laughter had subsided, he would say, " When I first met Miss Manie, I felt like I could eat her alive. After I married her, I wished like Hell that I had!"

Our family was a treasure chest of anecdotes, so I never ran out of a way to get a chuckle from my mother. What we thought was funny would have been silly to some people. But we had an attachment to the principals in our stories, so they didn't seem silly to us.

When I was a youngster, I spent summers with Mother's parents. The mailbox was a mile from the house and Granddaddy and I would walk to get the mail. His bait to get me to walk with him was that we would "crack a few jokes" as we walked and waited for the mail. He was full of simple country humor and I loved every minute of it! I guess Mother and I inherited his passion for a good story. He was a talker and a good storyteller.

One of our stories had to do with both of my grandfathers. They were as different as night and day. My father's father was a man of few words and spoke only when spoken to. After my mother and father were married, her parents came to visit his parents. The two old men were walking around the farm. Granddaddy T was asking a thousand questions and Granddaddy A was giving short, concise answers. Granddaddy T made the mistake of asking a question a second time. He said that the silence was deafening, then the other old man said, "I told you one time." He spoke in a very gruff voice and for the first time in his life Granddaddy T was speechless! But he told the story until his last days on Earth and Mother and I were left with the legacy.

Even when Mother's stories would get confused, she still told them as if she knew that every word was correct. I found that if I corrected her, she would become frustrated and forget where she was in the story. So I just let the chips fall where they may and everything was just fine. It really didn't make one bit of difference, because I knew every story by heart and she was enjoying telling her new version.

I could go on forever with our little stories. There was the time that Grandma's brother threw the croquet mallet the length of the court and killed Granddaddy's best rooster...and the one about Aunt Alma and my moneymaking machine...Granddaddy and the first traffic light he ever saw...Grandma and her hymn-singing and her motorcycle ride ...and Daddy and the block of ice. I won't bore you with narrative, but can assure you that we relived those and more many times in those four-plus years I was taking care of Mother.

Not everybody will be able to use this type of interchange to stimulate the one being cared for. Everybody has a different sense of humor. Some victims are past the point of being able to keep a story straight or to understand the gist of what's being said. Regardless, I feel that just simple conversation is helpful. A human voice has its own magic. Silence can be devastating. Even for those parked in a fog bank, the human experience is extremely important. All this has no scientific value, but I know that in my case, Mother responded. I felt that if I could preserve what quality of life she had left, then I was doing my job.

Chapter Twelve

Something's Wrong With The Furnace

Caregivers, you have to do what you think is best regardless of what people think.
You are in a better position to know your finances, the needs of the person for whom you are caring, and what you need personally.

Whoever said, "When it rains, it pours," really knew what they were talking about! It seems that bad luck begets bad luck, and my second winter in Virginia was a traumatic experience. Keeping warm was paramount in my book of things to do. I am a very warm-natured creature and when it drops below 70 degrees I become an inanimate object.

Mother had heated with oil for years. When we moved in to the house back in 1941, our first several years were spent with the mess associated with a coal furnace. After the war ended, the furnace was converted to oil and was the method of heating from then on. The old converted furnace was replaced with a real oil furnace when it had outlived its usefulness. It was in the house when I came back. Mother had a contract with the Oil Company: in the spring of each year the serviceman came out, cleaned the furnace and checked it for problems. He was the bearer of bad news. It needed so much work that a new furnace was the only alternative. We were living on a budget so tight that the routine daily needs put a squeeze on us, so I had no idea where a new furnace was coming from.

Then the next boot dropped! The week before, I had "stuck" the oil tank to measure the contents and it showed we had about a third of a tank left. For some reason I rechecked it after the serviceman had come and we had an empty tank. It didn't take a genius to figure out that the tank had sprung a leak and we had lost all the oil. It was a buried tank and a new law made the replacement even more costly. The reason for the law was to prevent from happening what had just happened to us. Old tanks were leaking oil into the aquifer and polluting drinking water. We had unintentionally added to the problem. This brought on a state of depression that made the Blue Funk seem like a picnic! I had no idea what I was going to do. Fortunately, it was late spring and the weather was pleasant enough to get by with just a light sweater. I had a summer to solve my problems. I was very thankful that it hadn't happened earlier in the year.

Even though it was spring, we would have some damp days. I would start a fire in the fireplace so that Mother didn't catch a cold. This took the dampness out of the living room, but dampness prevailed in the rest of the house. Mother would feel the radiator and try to adjust the thermostat. When the furnace didn't come on, she would tell me that something was wrong with it. I explained to her that we were out of oil and she would tell me that she would have to order more. I agreed and she forgot and all was well until she felt the radiator again. This went on until summer came and the hot, steamy Tidewater climate set in.

Then it was fan time. Mother had never enjoyed the frivolity of air conditioning. She had three or four of those hand fans that you used to get with the Funeral Home ad on the back and she used them to stir a breeze. She also lost them regularly. I spent many summer days hunting her fans. She would lay them down and walk away from them. She also had an electric oscillating fan that she bought when we moved in years ago. It had been knocked off its perch onto the floor many times and was warped out of shape. It was very noisy. My friend Jane gave me a box fan that she wasn't using, but it never replaced the old oscillator as far as Mother was concerned.

But back to the problem that I was facing concerning heat for the winter. I started weighing possibilities and came up with one I felt was worth investigating. The basement was completed now and it was in the corner of the house where the furnace room was located. I saw that I could go through the brick foundation and take a stovepipe to the chimney that served the furnace. Maybe I could put a wood stove in the basement and heat the house with wood. But where could I get enough wood to last through each winter? I started querying people and found that if I cut and hauled it, there would be quite a bit available simply by moving fallen trees and branches for people. Winter's ice took a toll on trees in that area. Also, one of my neighbors told me that there was fallen timber on his father's farm and I was welcome to move it. Jane had a wood stove in her house; she agreed to share wood from her farm if I would help her cut and split the wood. She had a chain saw and she gave me one as a gift out of the kindness of her heart. So the wood didn't seem to be a problem and it would be great exercise...which I could certainly use!

Now came the chore of locating a stove that would take big enough logs so that it could be banked and last through the night. The Richmond area had a great little paper called "The Trading Post". People could place an ad for free and only be billed if the item sold. I started scouring it for wood stoves of the proper size and price. I saw immediately that the price would be less than a tenth the cost of replacing the oil heat. Quite a few weeks went by and nothing showed up that was even worth calling about. Then it happened. A stove appeared that sounded exactly like what I needed. I called and got directions. It was quite a distance away, so I asked Perry to keep an eye on Mother and I headed out in the van.

Finally I arrived in the little farm town where the lady who had the stove lived, but I couldn't find the road she told me to take. I called again for directions. The number that she had given me was her place of work, close by. She led me down a long, winding dirt road for what seemed to be an eternity. We went into a shed away from the house and there was a custom-built monster of a wood stove. It was constructed of heavy-gauge steel that would last a lifetime. No telling what it had cost new. Looked to me like it weighed a ton and when I tried to lift it I wasn't far from right. But she was a big farm girl and assured me that we could handle it. Somehow I believed her, although I wasn't sure how.

She had me back the van up to the porch. Then she opened the stove door and started taking the firebricks out. We stacked them in the van and I could see that we had removed about fifty pounds of weight. I also saw that I was going to have to find a source for firebricks. Several of them badly needed replacing. She got on one side and I took the other and we walked the stove…first one side, then the other…out of the shed and across the porch to the van. She got a piece of plywood and made a bridge from the porch to the van. We lifted the front onto the bridge, then she found a large piece of pipe. Lifting the back of the stove and plywood up slightly, she slid the pipe under it. We used the edge of the porch as a fulcrum and the pipe as a lever and literally slid the stove, bridge and all, into the van. Farm girls know all about science!

Next, she went into another part of the shed and came out with enough good stove pipe so that I wouldn't have to buy anything but a few elbows. She also gave me a metal pad that goes under stoves to protect floors. My search in *The Trading Post* had really paid off. Now I had a really nice stove and only two things ahead of me that I wasn't looking forward to. One was a long drive back to Mother's house. The other was a very heavy stove that I had to get out of the van and down the steps into the basement. I paid the lady, thanked her, and off I went. After watching her in action, I knew that with a little ingenuity I could get the job done. My ego wouldn't let me stop until the stove was in the basement.

I got home in time for dinner and just left the stove in the van, watched a little TV, and got a good night's sleep. Perry had checked on Mother several times. She was just sitting in her rocker, either watching TV or gazing out of the window. She didn't even seem to know that I had been gone. Out of sight, out of mind!

Bright and early the next morning, I backed the van up to the basement steps and started the difficult task of moving the stove into its final resting place. I didn't ask Perry to help because he had a bad back and I like to work by myself when I really don't know what I'm doing. There was a space a little larger than the stove at the top of the steps, almost the same height as the van floor. I had two ten-foot two-by-fours that fit perfectly from the top step to the landing at the bottom. I had half a sheet of heavy plywood that fit on top of the two-by-fours, forming a ramp. Using a pipe lever like we had used to load the stove, I worked the plywood and stove from the van slowly out of the back door and onto the landing. It took quite awhile because I had to stop and rest frequently. And I had to answer the same question over and over, because Mother kept coming onto the porch to see what was going on. Finally I got the heavy mass onto the landing without hurting myself or breaking anything. The next stage would be the hardest and most dangerous.

I tied a heavy rope around the stove and looped it around my trailer hitch on the van. I knew that the weight of the stove would carry it down my temporary ramp once I got the stove onto the ramp. I could lower it down the ramp with the rope. Only fools and egotists attempt things like this!

Since I qualified in both cases, I started working the stove onto the ramp, staying behind the stove in case it got away. Luckily, it didn't and I successfully lowered the monster to the bottom landing. Now I moved the plywood the lady had given me onto the basement floor and located the metal pad where the stove would sit. The plywood and the pad were close to the same thickness, so if I could slide stove and plywood across the floor, I could work the stove onto the pad. After much ado, I got the stove into place and issued a loud sigh of relief! Let me tell you, it is much easier to write about it than it actually was to do it!

Now that I knew that I had a stove, I could remove the furnace. I had to do this after Mother was in bed because she would have driven me crazy asking questions. I got it disconnected during the day and moved it out in one night. I disassembled it after it was out in the yard and used parts for various things, including giving Perry some of the good working parts to use as backup for his furnace.

After the furnace was removed, I opened a hole through the wall from basement to furnace room for the stovepipe. Then I connected the pipe and the stove was ready for use. It was mid-summer and I didn't want to build a fire to check the stove out, so I was really spinning the roulette wheel and gambling that all was well. I knew that if it didn't work, my daughters would help me buy a furnace, but I wanted to do it my way and not have to depend on them. I got that streak of independence from the lady for whom I was now caring!

A neighbor down the street had asked Perry if he knew of anybody who wanted a used air conditioner air handler. He had replaced his system and wanted to give it away. I jumped on it and mounted it on top of the stove, connecting simple ductwork to a few strategically-placed registers that I installed in the floor. I rigged it so that the fan only came on when the air temperature in the box was warm, so that it didn't blow cold air into the house. Thank God for my engineering schooling! Many of the things I did I wouldn't have had the slightest notion about without the schooling. I now had a system that would move the heat from the stove into the house with very little use of power. So far, so good.

Now I started collecting wood. I constructed a woodshed out back and started filling it with wood that people gave me. There was a lot of manual labor involved...cutting and splitting oak isn't a picnic. I enjoyed it, though, because the exercise was good and I couldn't afford to become a couch potato. I also found it to be educational. I had been in Florida for so long I didn't know which wood was good firewood and which wasn't. I asked many questions and got many answers. Some were correct, and some I later found to be bogus when the wood just lay in the stove and gave off little heat.

Fall came. The big test was upon me. I had gotten new firebricks and had a clean stove ready for blastoff. Lo and behold, it worked like a champ. It drew well and I could control it with the built-in dampers. The chimney worked great and so did the air handler. It waited until the stove surface got hot, then started to blow warm air through the floor registers. The heat in the basement warmed the wooden floor above and further transferred heat into the house. An additional plus was that the exposed stovepipe in the furnace room (which I had now converted into a utility room) heated the kitchen when the door was ajar. The only negative was that you could smell wood burning, but it was the same as having a fire in the fireplace.

Mother started her parade back and forth from her rocker to the thermostat. Regardless of the room temperature, if the radiator wasn't warm she would say that there was something wrong with the furnace and go make an adjustment. I had the thermostat disconnected but left it so she could fool with it.

I had to do something to make her think that everything was all right so she wouldn't wear herself out making her trips. My uncle had built very nice radiator covers with metal screens in the front. This is what Mother would feel. I got a small ceramic electric heater that was thermostatically controlled. I mounted it in the cover so that it would warm the screen and also help heat the area where she sat, since that was next to a window and outside wall. It was quiet and very efficient. You could hardly see the power meter move when it came on. It did the trick!

People kidded me about my source of heat, but I had the last laugh. The winter before Mother passed was a really bad one for Virginia. During one of the ice-snow storms 750,000 people were without power for a whole week. We were included, along with our neighbors. Furnaces require power to control the thermostat and the carburetor. Heat pumps couldn't work. But the guy that had been kidded about his wood heat was warm as toast. He who laughs last laughs best! We had to use candles at night and Mother retired earlier than usual, but that old wood stove in the basement kept on working. Without power, the air handler couldn't work, but I took the cover off it so the heat could still rise up through the registers and all was well.

Caregivers, you have to do what you think is best regardless of what people think. You are in a better position to know your finances, the needs of the person for whom you are caring, and what you need personally. What I did was a bit bizarre in most people's minds, but it worked for me. You handle the situation; don't let the situation control you!

Chapter Thirteen

Padlock The Freezer Door And Out With The Kitchen Cabinet Shelves

You have to learn to cope. I developed patience by ignoring things that I could not control. I kept telling myself that certain things really didn't matter.

No cook stove. No furnace. An attic stairway screwed shut. Now two more inconveniences were upon me. Imagine living for four years with the refrigerator freezer padlocked! Mother's memory was costing money and making it impossible for me to keep her weight under control. Her recreation was taking things from the freezer to thaw, because she thought that mealtime was all the time. She would also rearrange things, moving items from the freezer to the refrigerator and vice versa. Besides that, on a number of occasions I went into the kitchen and was greeted by the gaping mouth of an open freezer door. She would open it to take something out and then be distracted, walking away and leaving the door open.

She had a real love of ice cream and couldn't remember that she had just had a serving five minutes ago. It did no good to say anything, because she simply didn't understand. So I put a hasp on the freezer door and locked it shut. I had to unlock it every time I needed to get things out, but those things sure did last longer.

I had switched from ice cream to frozen yogurt to help with the cholesterol and weight problems, but even that didn't help if one consumed too much. Mother enjoyed this delicious dessert so much that I had no intention of not having it available for her. I suspected that she was making many trips to the freezer when I kept finding spoon trails in the yogurt box. Mother would eat out of the box very neatly so there were no gouges like the ones I made. She would make many trips a day and peel off a thin layer. The crowning blow came when she ate a half-gallon in one day! Padlock, here we come! I didn't want to deprive her of one of her few extravagances, but I couldn't afford to buy enough to supply that kind of intake. And it simply wasn't good for her. So I had no choice but to block her entrance. If you are a caregiver, you understand. If you become one you will get the picture quickly.

After I put the lock on, I could hear her rattling it, trying to get the freezer open. She would tell me that "they" had locked the freezer and she didn't know how she was going to fix meals. I rationed her frozen yogurt and made sure that she had an ample amount each day. I would have to hide things that I was thawing for meals because she would move them or put them in the refrigerator if they were left on the kitchen counter. She thought that it was her responsibility to keep the kitchen straight. I also had to hide the key to the lock in a place convenient for me, but hard for her to find. Being without a range and oven wasn't nearly as inconvenient as this was. You probably don't realize how many times you go into a freezer, especially if you don't have an ice dispenser in the door. Every time you want an iced drink...into the freezer you go. It's almost an involuntary reaction and when you run into a roadblock you become very agitated. Try it and see.

The frozen yogurt wasn't the only thing in the refrigerator that fell prey to the phantom snacker. My friend Jane brought me a birthday cake. I put it in the refrigerator to enjoy later and went out to work in the yard and on the outside of the house. I was out for about three hours because I got engrossed in my projects. When I went in to fix lunch, the empty cake plate was on the kitchen counter. Yes, I said empty! Mother had eaten the whole thing. She didn't even leave me a crumb. I guess she thought that it was her birthday, so she could eat her cake.

The kitchen had been Mother's major domain for many years. It was her natural stomping grounds. So she felt obligated to do her duty and tidy it up. The next problem I faced was not only frustrating, it was dangerous for her. I mentioned earlier that she had fallen from the kitchen counter onto her head several years ago. I also said that the doctor had given orders for her not to climb stairs without help, because her medication affected her balance. Well, I don't know how many times I entered the kitchen to find her up on the counter moving things around on the cabinet shelves. There were two cabinets, with canned goods and other cooking necessities on one side, dishes, glasses, and the like on the other. She would move things from the top shelf to the bottom one time, then move them back the next time.

For the most part, Mother was very docile and easy to get along with. She would do what she was asked and not question why…except for having to get down from the counter. On several occasions I actually had to lift her down, with her banging me on the head with her fist. Let me tell you, for an old lady, she packed quite a wallop!

So what could I do to make the lady of the house stay off the counter? I reasoned that if there were fewer shelves, there would be less need for arranging. And if the shelves were reachable from the floor there would be no need to climb on the counter. There were about five removable shelves on both sides. So I removed three from each cabinet. I left just the necessary dishes, glasses and such in one cabinet and put the balance in the attic. That had to be done when Mother was on one her garden strolls, so she wouldn't try to follow me into the attic. Since there were only two of us and we certainly didn't throw any dinner parties, many things could be moved from that cabinet.

Several years before, my friend Jane had a fire in her house that required a major renovation. She had salvaged most of the counters and cabinets from her kitchen and bath. She told me that I could have what I wanted, so I got a cabinet that I could mount on one wall at eye level. It was over the microwave and I used it to store my microwave cooking utensils. Since it was associated with the microwave, Mother steered clear. Even if she had wanted to move things around, the cabinet was low enough to make climbing unnecessary.

The other cabinet posed a bigger problem. I decided that my best bet was to make more trips to the grocer and buy fewer canned goods on each trip. There were also two cabinets under the counter. I jammed them full of things from the top cabinet. This served a second purpose. Now Mother could rearrange things from bottom to top and back without climbing. I felt that the more active I could keep her without putting her in danger's way, the better off both of us would be. The drawback was that every time I needed something, the hunt was on! She also had drawers to tidy up, so I never knew where I would find a knife, folk or spoon, let alone a cooking utensil. She meticulously moved things to places where you would never think to look. I often wonder how many times that kitchen had been redone before I came to stay.

Soon after I arrived and before I had to disconnect the stove, I had built a pullout that went next to the stove. I cut out a big rooster since Mother had several ceramic roosters on the back of the stove. I made it so utensils could be hung on hooks on the rooster and pans could be stored in the lower compartment. The unit was on casters and was pulled out to access the pans. Mother never bothered these things, because she wouldn't pull the thing out and it was foreign to her kitchen. After the stove was disabled, I left these items in the pullout. It opened up storage in the cabinets and allowed me to move more canned goods to the lower cabinet. Mother liked to look at the rooster, but never removed a spoon or spatula.

When Mother got bored from rocking and looking out the window, she headed either to her room or the kitchen to straighten things out. She loved to decorate and was very artistic. One fall she started decorating the kitchen table with fallen maple leaves. I had two TV tables that I used for our meals in the living room, since it was easier than getting her to the table. We watched TV and ate and it worked out just fine. From time to time relatives would come and bring food. We would get real classy and use the dining room table. That pleased Mother; she thought she was entertaining as she used to do so often. She was a gracious hostess and we had many great meals at that table when I was growing up.

The kitchen table sat empty; she decided it needed a centerpiece. The big maple in the back yard dropped tons of leaves. When Mother made a trip into the yard she came back with a handful of leaves. She arranged them neatly in the center of the table. Then the pile started to grow! We had several large pines in the yard and they contributed pine cones. Every trip produced more leaves or cones and they went onto the table. As it grew, it became an attraction for visitors and that pleased Mother. I decided to leave it and see where it ended. I could have removed the leaves and controlled the spread, but I just let it grow. Before the leaves had stopped falling and dead winter set in, the table was completely covered.

I left the leaves for quite some time. They got rearranged over and over. It was almost like looking at a kaleidoscope. Every time I went into the kitchen a new pattern had evolved. Alzheimer's didn't seem to impair Mother's artistic ability in the least. I imagine that at some point it would have had an impact. But I was fortunate. In the spring there were flowers to arrange. Even if it was only a handful of dandelions, they were put in a vase and carefully adjusted for stem length and greenery. She worked slowly, but the outcome was always visually satisfying. Actually, Mother would go into a garden full of flowers and come in with dandelions. I don't know why she wouldn't pick the flowers and will never know. I asked several times and she would tell me that no flowers were blooming. That was the result of the three-minute window I talked about earlier. Anyway, in the fall there were leaves and pine cones. For what more could a fellow ask!

Researchers say that Alzheimer's disease includes any or all of the following detectable symptoms. The most noticeable, and usually first to develop, is memory impairment. This can be combined with language disturbance, impaired motor functions, failure to recognize or identify objects, and the inability to plan or organize. Mother's memory was definitely impaired. She had no language disturbance, except that sometimes she could not find the right word to express a thought. I didn't consider that a symptom because that happens to me frequently. Her motor functions deteriorated with time. She never had a problem recognizing or identifying objects. And although her planning ability was nil, she sure could organize those flowers and leaves.

Caregivers need patience or they will never make it through the ordeal. You have to learn to cope. I developed patience by ignoring things that I could not control. I kept telling myself that certain things really didn't matter. I tried to stay focused on trying to keep Mother from inadvertently hurting herself. At one point in my life, those leaves would have gone out as fast as they were brought in. But I kept telling myself that they were serving a purpose, so I let Mother create her table art. I only know what worked for me. Each situation is different, so I don't think anyone can give particular advice. If you are thrust into the role of caregiver, just be patient and you will make it.

Chapter Fourteen

Grocery Bags Make A Fine Suitcase

*I was always anxious at night
and my sleep wasn't as restful as I needed it to be.
Sleep without rest is not very useful.*

Usually when Mother went to bed she slept soundly. She would get up quietly several times to use the bathroom, but didn't awaken me. There were, however, occasions when she would do things completely out of reason, so I learned to sleep with one ear open, so to speak. I always worried about what would happen if she decided to go outside in the middle of the night. I tried to be aware of where she was if she wasn't in bed. Usually if she missed her naps during the day and got overtired, she would have a bad night. On occasion she would rearrange her room or the kitchen late at night. Perry reported that he saw the light in her room go on and off repeatedly late at night. She kept her door closed so I usually wasn't aware of it. Sometimes I did see the light shining under her door. Fortunately she didn't actually go outside at night, but the concern was always there.

When I would hear her rambling at night, I would get up and distract her and talk her back to bed. Several times she would knock on my door, which I kept ajar, and say strange things. It was obvious that she was confused. It took some doing to convince her that whatever she thought was happening really wasn't. One night she told me that there were a bunch of guys with motorcycles living next door and they were coming and going all the time. Actually, Perry did have a motorcycle when they moved in next door, but that was several years prior to her concern and he had sold it. I would take her to her bedroom window and show her that there were only two cars and no motorcycles next door. She would say that she guessed they had gone. I'd settle her down and she'd go back to sleep. I am a person who needs my sleep. This light sleeping with many interruptions took its toll. Although I had never been able to nap during the day, I developed the ability and tried to snooze during one of her daytime naps. It became a habit and now I take a daily nap. I guess I'm becoming an old man!

One night, Mother knocked on my door and said that "they" were coming to pick her up. She said the doorbell was ringing and wanted me to see who it was. Of course, if the bell had rung, I would have heard it, but I obliged her and went to the front door. By the time I got back she had forgotten all about it and was tucked into bed again.

I never knew when my sleep would be interrupted and it was very frustrating. There was no cure for the problem. I believe that dreams had a lot to do with it. When a dream awakens you, sometimes it appears to be real. If your mental gears aren't meshing properly, I'm sure that you could believe most anything was happening. "They" could really be at the door!

I understand that many Alzheimer's sufferers get up in the middle of the night and leave the house. My friend Harold did, so I was told. That was in the back of my mind for four long years. We lived in a small community where many people knew Mother, but many didn't. With people moving in and out all the time, and with her being out of circulation for almost ten years, if she got lost I would really have had a problem finding her. Although she only got lost once, and that was in the middle of the day, it still worried me. So I tried to keep tabs on her even when I was asleep. I'm not trying to scare present and future caregivers, just offering a word of caution. It seems that when people with Alzheimer's get lost, they become more confused and that amplifies the problem. In normal circumstances, Mother knew her street name and house number, but the one time that she wandered, she couldn't remember them. If the lady who found her hadn't known who she was, it would have been a real problem.

I had to learn as I went. When I became a caregiver I hardly knew what Alzheimer's disease was. I had heard about it on TV and read a few articles in magazines and newspapers, but if you are not directly concerned it doesn't sink in. When I first came to live with her, Mother was far more active, both during the day and at night. It was her house and I felt like a visitor. I could hear her rattling around in the kitchen at night and thought she knew what she was doing. It turned out that the ice cream in the freezer was one of the attractions. But she also did her share of rearranging dishes and such at night also. After several of her escapades, like getting me up to greet "them" at the front door, I started getting up and checking on her. It aggravated her to be constantly spied on and she would say a few caustic words. I tried to make it look as if I just happened to get up. I'd get drinks of water, or check to make sure the porch light was turned off or that the door was locked. I became a pretty good actor, even though the deceit bothered me. Here I was checking on a lady in her own house that she had occupied for over fifty years. This was my mother! It really took some mental conditioning to make myself realize that she was now the child and that I was literally the parent. I was learning what Alzheimer's disease was all about.

One night I was aroused by a ruckus coming from Mother's room. She slept with the door shut, but she was obviously into something. I knocked on the door. She had a very worried look on her face. The bed was littered with her sewing paraphernalia, collected over many years. She had a three-tier sewing basket that opened two ways, exposing six compartments. Every compartment was empty and the contents were on the bed. I asked what she was looking for and she had forgotten. She was tired and when she wore herself out she became confused. She couldn't go back to bed because of the mess on top of it. It took me nearly an hour to get the stuff back into the basket in a haphazard fashion. One of her distractions was sorting through the buttons, ribbons, elastic, pins, snaps, rickrack, zippers, iron-on patches, thread, empty bobbins, and other very valuable gadgets and gewgaws she had stored away. I knew that my main job was to clear the bed and get her back in it. Finally I could return to my very interrupted sleep, knowing that she had exhausted herself and would probably sleep until sunup.

Another night I was really tired when I went to bed and fell into a deep sleep. I was startled by cabinet doors banging and could tell that Mother was on another tear. I jumped up and found her in the bathroom. There were about two-dozen paper grocery bags sitting on the floor full of everything you can imagine. Mother was emptying the medicine cabinet into a bag. She was fully dressed, although she seldom got out of her gown and robe anymore. She had cleaned out her dresser and had clothes piled into grocery bags. I asked what was going on and she said that Aunt Bebe (her sister) was coming to get her and she had to be ready for a long trip. Her sister had been in an assisted living facility for many years and hadn't driven in an even longer time.

This night I really didn't know how to handle the situation. Mother had worked herself into a frenzy. As long as she could see her stuff in those bags, it was hard to distract her. I had to do some quick thinking. I told Mother that I thought I heard Aunt Bebe at the front door and asked her to check. When she left I hurried and piled all of those bags into my room and shut the door. Then I went into the living room where Mother was sitting in her rocker. I sat on the couch for a few minutes, looked at my watch and told her it was time to go to bed. She had completely forgotten about the expected visitor and quietly went back to bed. It took me several hours to get back to sleep because I was having an adrenaline rush like I had never experienced before! The next day I spent most of the morning emptying grocery bags back into drawers and cabinets. I laughed to myself, thinking that I was unpacking Mother's expensive luggage.

Whenever it stormed I could count on a lot of moving around...day or night. Mother went from window to window, onto the side porch, down to the back door, and became very nervous. She worried about the big maple tree falling on the house and I had a real problem getting her to settle down. Central Virginia has some real strong windstorms and thunder and lightening. I had lived in the Tampa Bay area, the lightning capitol of the World, for forty years, but I do believe that our part of Virginia held a very close second place! She checked windows to make sure that they were closed and forgot which ones she had checked. So it was a constant prowl from window to window and no rest for the weary.

Some of her concern had a fair basis. The house had storm windows. She had hired some inept "Mr. Fix-it" to caulk around the windows. Whenever a hard rain came, the water was held inside some of the storm windows and drained into the house onto the hardwood floors. The floor in the room I used was ruined. One of my first tasks was to correct the problem. Storm windows have what is called weep holes to let the water that gets in drain out. They had been caulked closed! But Mother didn't seem to forget about the water coming in, and couldn't remember that I had fixed the problem. So rain wasn't my favorite gift of nature.

As the years passed, the frequency of the nocturnal disturbances decreased. I tried to make sure that Mother got two naps a day and the duration of the naps increased with time. I thought that the more quiet rest Mother got, the less active she was at night. I have nothing but supposition to back this up, but I do know that if she got tired or stressed, I could bet on a bad night. It seemed that, as the disease progressed, the more willing she was to sit and rock. But I never stopped worrying about what might happen. I was always anxious at night and my sleep wasn't as restful as I needed it to be. Sleep without rest is not very useful.

What in the world went on in that house before I came back to stay? How did my mother avoid hurting herself? I have wondered that so many times after I found out how her life was spent. And the writing of this book brings things back into focus, making me wonder even more. People who knew Mother, like our relatives and her close friends, had no idea what she did when nobody was around. I imagine that there are many people in the same condition and living in the same circumstances all over, everywhere. I now live alone and can see how habits develop and become a way of life. I pray that I am never afflicted with this dreadful disease.

Chapter Fifteen

Would You Please Wind My Watch?

Mother was obsessed with time. She was continually looking at her watch, asking me to wind it, and asking me the time. This obsession with time is a mystery to me to this day.

Mother was obsessed with time. She was continually looking at her watch, asking me to wind it, and asking me the time. For somebody lost in space, this obsession with time is a mystery to me to this day. I acted as if I was winding that watch dozens of times some days. It was usually correct and wound tight as a tick, but she always thought it was wrong. She would check it against the TV when they gave the time and she would go into the kitchen and look at the clock over the refrigerator. I always wondered why she trusted that clock as opposed to her watch. But she did, and if they said the same thing, all was well.

For years, the way people checked for the correct time was to call the telephone operator. Although now there is a number to dial to check time, Mother never changed her method and she kept calling the operator. She dialed "O" and asked for the time many times a day and at night. I heard her late at night checking time. I had to install a phone in my room and had a FAX machine and answering machine. Calls would come in for me and I'd never get the messages, so I turned the ringer off on the phone that she always used. But she could still make calls. She could hear the phone ring in my room, but she figured that it was a different phone and never tried to answer. I had the same problem with the mail. I had to keep an eagle eye out because the mailbox was in Mother's line of vision from her rocker. I had to make sure that I got it before she did, or I'd never see it. This happened to several bills when I first started my caregiver job. I had to make phone calls and explain the problem to avoid credit problems.

    I finally decided to buy her a quartz watch with a battery so that she wouldn't have to be winding all of the time. I didn't realize that Mother wouldn't remember that it didn't need winding. She kept asking me to wind it. She would twist the setting knob thinking she was winding. And she kept her telephone vigil and her trips to the kitchen clock. I would pretend to wind it after I gave up trying to explain about the battery and that it was keeping time without winding. I can't explain the obsession with time since her day consisted of getting up in the morning, passing the day away, and going to bed at night. Daylight got her up and darkness sent her to bed, but she always wanted to know the time. It probably was habit established many years ago. My oldest daughter refuses to wear a watch or live on a time-oriented schedule because it crimps her artistic lifestyle. She is probably more sane because of it.

    Many times, when Mother would start looking at her watch and looking out the window, I used to kid her. When she was a young girl, my Aunt Alma lived in Southside, Vifginia, in a very small village named Bracey. She visited quite often until she moved to teach school. When Mother started looking out the window, I would tell her that the bus to Bracey was probably late, but it should be here soon. She would pout and say that she didn't want to go to Bracey! Then she would laugh and tell me about her visits when she was a girl. She could recount things that you would expect to be gone from memory by that time. She was very close to Aunt Alma and that might be why the memories lingered. Of course I had no way of knowing the accuracy of her stories, but it was interesting to hear how times have changed. Drawing water from a well... washing clothes in a tin tub and scrub board... riding in a horse and buggy...sleeping in a feather bed... using an outhouse for the necessities of life: I had done some of those things, but it is hard to believe that those were parts of daily life and taken for granted. Uncle Roy had one of the first cars in that part of the country and that was Mother's first car ride. She smiled widely when she told about that ride! The bus to Bracey never came, but Mother's concern about time never stopped either.

Since I've been writing this, I decided to pay attention to the number of times I look at my watch in a day. I get up at a certain time and the first thing I look at is my watch. I walk four miles a day at two different times. I walk at four miles an hour and time it with a stopwatch. I eat lunch and dinner at approximately the same time each day. I have a favorite bedtime and usually am very punctual. All of this is managed by looking at my watch. You may be surprised at how many times you check the time. It's almost an involuntary action. Try it. I'll bet that it will blow your mind. Now imagine that you have no point of reference for knowing whether the watch is right or not. We use the sun's position, routine happenings in our daily life, TV and radio, and many more events to know if the time is in the ballpark. Mother had lost those points of reference. Her watch was her gospel and she wanted it to be right. She was in a time void and therefore time became an obsession. When I say time void, an example is her age. She was 84 years old when I arrived. She had four birthdays while I was there. But in her mind she was 84 all that time. In fact, although she was almost 89 when she passed, she bragged to visitors about being 84 and in perfect health!

Here again, this is just some more of my amateur analysis. I haven't found anything in print that actually verified my assumptions. I also don't know if other caregivers experience this time warp. Every case is different. All I know is that my mother wanted to be on time for whatever came along.

Chapter Sixteen

The Old Switch-The-Walking-Stick Trick

*Mother knew that something was wrong
with her memory, but really didn't understand
the problem. Sometimes she would say
that she wondered where she had been for years.*

When I was five or six years old, I received a wallop on my backside that stung like a hornet. It was from my Grandfather's walking cane. I had shut the car door on his favorite white Panama hat and it got torn. That walking cane came back to haunt me years later. Mother was unsteady on her feet and used Granddaddy's old cane to get around with. She kept it with her all the time, that is, except when it was lost. She would go into the backyard or in the garden, decide to do something like pull a weed or two, put the cane down and forget it. I don't know how many times I was summoned to find that old walking stick. It became a game with me. I kept a mental record of the many places where she had stowed it. The problem was that it totally unnerved her when it was gone. It now hangs on my living room wall as a constant reminder of the swat on the bottom and the many hours I spent searching for my nemesis.

I found it hanging on various limbs of trees in the yard, stuck down in tomato vines, on the low roof of my lawnmower shed, in high grass, hanging on a neighbor's fence...only to name a few places. Mother had a propensity for losing things. She had an opal ring that was her birthstone. She loved that ring and showed it to me almost every day. It was loose on her finger and she had wrapped tape around it to make it fit better. During the second year of my stay, it occurred to me that Mother hadn't showed me her ring lately. I asked her where it was. She came unglued! She had no idea where it was. It was gone.

I searched the house high and low but found no ring. Mother was in tears. I consoled her, but it didn't do much good. It is one of the few times that she displayed real emotion. Trying to get her to retrace her steps was impossible. I had no idea how long the ring had been gone and neither did she.

I got her to go with me out into the yard. It is hard to conceive, but she couldn't remember from one minute to the next what we were looking for. She got distracted with something in the garden and soon was headed back into the house. I decided to go buy a cheap metal detector. It was a waste of money. I searched the whole yard, front and back, but no ring. After several days the ring had disappeared from Mother's mind, but I really felt badly that I couldn't find it. It had little monetary value but was heaped with sentimentality. Since it was loose on her finger, I thought that it might have gone down the drain in either the kitchen or bathroom. I removed both goosenecks, but there was no ring. It was just simply gone.

Back to the walking cane. I decided to try an experiment. I was afraid that the walking cane would go the way of the opal ring, so I made an "outside cane" for Mother out of a hoe handle and another round piece of wood. I made a holder next to the back door and showed it to Mother. We discussed how she would leave the inside cane in the holder and use the outside cane in the yard. Then she was to switch when she came back. It worked sometimes...sometimes it didn't. She would forget to switch going out, or she would switch going out and forget on the way back. She continued to lose the canes, regardless of which one she had. On one occasion both sticks were carried out and lost! The two canes helped; on more times than not Mother would do it right. When I'd see her heading out back, I'd remind her to switch. Many times I had to exchange canes after she had made it back to her rocker.

There is a lot of morning dew in our part of Virginia. Mother would slip into a pair of boots when she went out in the wet. I put her cane exchange next to where the boots stayed. The boots always got taken off when she came back in, but the canes were a hit-or-miss proposition.

When I first moved back, Mother had an onion patch behind her shed. It wasn't well tended but she liked to dabble in the patch. She had a good supply of garden tools that had collected over the years. People would give her new things and she'd keep the old ones. Remember, her slogan was, "You never know when you'll need something." Well, while she was dabbling in her onion patch she lost a trowel. I searched and searched but never found it. A year later I dug the onion patch up and moved the shed. To my dismay the trowel never turned up and it was never seen again. It was her favorite trowel, but in a few days she totally forgot about it. Not many tools were misplaced, because as time went on Mother dabbled less and less. She would pull a few weeds and pick up a few sticks, but her gardening was at an end. It is so sad to see a person who was once so active simply give up. She never stopped talking about what she had to do in her yard and in her garden, but she never got around to doing it.

I never knew what was going to get lost next. Sometimes a pot from the kitchen would be carried out when Mother thought that she had to pick some vegetables. Invariably the pot would get left in the garden. She had a pair of kitchen shears that she used to cut flowers. I spent plenty of time hunting shears. One time they were gone for two days and turned up in her robe pocket! After that, when small things were misplaced, a shakedown was in order. Usually Mother would sheepishly pull the object out of a pocket. She knew that something was wrong with her memory, but really didn't understand the problem. Sometimes she would say that she wondered where she had been for years. It embarrassed her not to be able to remember, so I would make a "gloss-over" comment and bring up another subject.

Inside the house, one of the things she most commonly mislaid were her glasses. When she had her cataract removed she got two pairs. I kept one pair put away for just this kind of emergency. After she was able to see again, it was usually a real chore to find the others. She had secret places where she stowed things; to this day I don't think that I found them all. Sometimes they were just left behind a curtain or under her pillow, or any place where she had a reason to remove them. Since her vision without her glasses wasn't that great, she usually didn't get far before calling me for help. That localized the search and made it easier.

It takes infinite patience to be a caregiver. Sometimes you feel like screaming until your lungs hurt, but that helps nothing and upsets the person for whom you are caring. I was fortunate that Mother never lost her ability to recognize objects. She knew when her glasses were gone or that she couldn't find her shears. It would be terrible to have something lost and not have a clue what was missing! I really had plenty for which to be thankful.

Chapter Seventeen

Mentioning The Unmentionables

*My relatives were a great help
with the personal hygiene problem.
Mother loved the attention and it was
very much appreciated by me.*

The hardest part of my job was to make sure that Mother's personal hygiene needs were attended. Being a male kind of put a crimp in my style. I had to use many devious means and get help from family members to assure that these things were under control. She took care of most of her bathing, although it took forever and I would have to knock on the bathroom door to make sure that she was all right. Getting gowns changed so they could be washed was a big problem. I would lay out a clean gown in plain view when I knew that she was going to bathe. Then I would remind her when she went in and knock on the door to remind her again. I know that it annoyed her, but she would have worn the same gown forever if I didn't ride herd on the situation. Although she had enough gowns to wear a different one every day of the week, getting her into a new one was like pulling teeth. Her frugal streak kicked in: new gowns were kept for special occasions.

I said earlier that Mother made her own bed. The problem was that she never changed the sheets and pillowcases. I had to go in after she had made the bed, change the linen, and remake the bed while she was occupied with some distraction. I tried laying out the bedding but it never got on the bed. Sometimes she would actually put the stuff away! Since her time reference had become defective, days, weeks, and months were meaningless. I had to make sure that everything happened in certain time intervals. This had been a most meticulous woman who couldn't stand it when everything wasn't just right. Now she couldn't keep up with the simplest routine.

To keep her healthy I had to keep her regular. I made sure that she had plenty of fiber in her diet and insisted that she drink plenty of water. Prunes were a part of her diet. But I had no way of knowing if it was working, because Mother couldn't remember what had happened in the bathroom by the time that she got into her rocker. I devised a somewhat inaccurate method by using two rolls of toilet paper. Mine was hidden. I gauged usage by the decrease of paper on the roll. Non-scientific, but it did help me some. This may be crude talk, but I am trying to point out to future caregivers some of the pitfalls in store for you. On more occasions than not, Mother would forget to flush. I routinely checked the commode to make sure that she was doing her business. I was so afraid that she would become constipated and wouldn't know the difference, or that she would develop diarrhea and wouldn't tell me.

I discovered I wouldn't have to worry about that when one day she came to me and told me that she had a problem. She said that she couldn't go potty. I gave her a laxative and waited to see if it cleared the problem. Poor Mother had soon forgotten the laxative and came back to me with just the opposite problem. If it hadn't been so sad, it would have been funny. I had to be very careful with the laxative from then on. I increased her prune servings and hoped for the best.

I helped Mother wash her hair. We would wash it in the kitchen sink and put a towel around it until it dried. She had beautiful, natural curly hair that didn't need rolling or setting of any kind. When she was a young girl, her sister Bebe was very jealous of her curly hair. Aunt Bebe had hair as straight as a stick. Mother used to laugh and tell about the time that Aunt Bebe chased her around the house with a pair of scissors threatening to cut all her curls off. My aunt verified the story with a shy giggle.

My relatives were a great help with the personal hygiene problem. They would come and trim her fingernails and toenails, make sure that she was bathing properly, and brush her hair. Occasionally one of my cousins would wash her hair and trim it up for her. Mother loved the attention and it was very much appreciated by me. They would go through her underwear drawers and remove things that had become too badly worn. My cousin Carolyn would bring new things and make sure that the diaper situation was under control. I can never thank all of them enough for all of the help they gave. Everybody has a life of their own and in our society they are rushed too much to have any spare time for others. But my family made time and my hat goes off to them! I had more on my plate than I could handle and wouldn't have made it without their help.

Most caregivers will probably have to do even more than I had to do in caring for the bodily needs of their loved one. I hear all of the time about people having to bath and dress the patient. In many cases, they have to put the affected one on the commode and make sure that all functions are working. I am very thankful that my mother could do most of the things that we humans do daily. She was slow and would forget what she had and hadn't done, but she usually did what was necessary. I stood in constant fear that the situation would deteriorate and I had no idea what I would do. People suggested that I get a professional to come in occasionally, but when I checked prices I knew that there wasn't room in our budget for that.

I was adamant that I would not put Mother in a care facility unless I had no other way out. My prayers were answered and I was able to care for her to the end. Even though she was lost in a fog I know that she was pleased that I could keep her at home. In her mind she was caring for me. I was a guest in her home and I was still her little Bobby! All that matters is that her health and welfare were never compromised. I can look back on it as just another challenge in life that I got through somehow.

Chapter Eighteen

That Dreaded Bedroom Door

Why should a bedroom door be such a problem? Because I never knew what I would find behind that door, that's why.

Why should a bedroom door be such a problem? Because I never knew what I would find behind that door, that's why. It was inevitable that one day I would have to face the reality of death. That was one subject I still have trouble dealing with. We fear what we don't understand, and the transition from this life to an after-life is very troubling to me.

I knew that I would probably find Mother when she passed and I wasn't sure that I could handle it. I also knew that life is so fragile that I could go before her. I couldn't find a place in the equation for that. I accept death, but it is such an unknown that I don't like to face it. I understand that the "child" in me was taking over. My "adult" abandoned me and let me fend for myself. I haven't changed one bit and probably will never change.

I don't like funerals. I positively refuse to stare into a coffin. The last time I did that, I was seven years old and my grandfather was lying there. I decided at that very early age that it is better to remember the living rather than the dead. When my first wife died she was living with my daughter, Holly. I went over with my older daughter, Kiaralinda. A friend of the family got bent out of shape when I refused to go into the bedroom and see Beverly. (Yes, I was married to two Beverlys!) We had been divorced several years but were on friendly terms. I chose to remember her as I had known her during our twenty-seven years together rather than see her in a state that I could not understand.

So Mother's bedroom door was a monument to a fear that I could not dismiss.

Our bedroom doors were at each end of a very short hallway. At Mother's end was the doorway into the dining room and the rest of the house. I had to pass her door to get out of my room and into the rest of the world. She kept the door shut when she was sleeping, but when more time had passed than I thought should, I had to force myself to crack the door and look in. It was like pulling teeth! Mother was a very quiet sleeper, hardly breathing as she slept. Many times in my four-year tour my heart skipped a beat when I opened that door. On a number of occasions, I actually had to feel a pulse in her neck to make sure that all was well. That usually awakened her and interrupted her rest. Nobody could tell me how else to handle it, so I kept checking with hope against hope that all was well.

As time went on, Mother's naps would last longer and longer, so I had to check more often. I realize that it was rather morbid continually to expect the worse, but I really couldn't help it.

It was a great relief when I passed the door and heard Mother shuffling around in her room. I didn't know what she was up to, but at least I knew that she was up. I guess that in the back of my mind I remembered that she had found Daddy when he died and had completely buried it in her subconscious. I didn't want to be alone when the time came, but had no way of assuring that somebody would be on hand to help me get through the trauma.

The door had become such a tender spot for me that I had actually considered putting another opening from my room to the living room. After thinking it through, I realized that I would still have to keep checking on Mother anyway, so why go to the trouble. I simply had to come to grips with reality and not try to circumvent the facts of life. I don't like confrontation or anything that brings mental anguish. I guess that's the coward coming out. But the truth is that there are certain things that just can't be avoided and have to be faced, regardless of the scar it leaves.

If you are a caregiver or are called upon later to be one, this is something that you should consider. You need to try to figure out how you are going to handle the situation. I'm sure that I'm in the minority when it comes to handling the passing of life. People in many professions work with it on a daily basis. Everybody in the medical profession seems to take death for granted. People work in many facets of the funeral business. Firemen and policemen handle death as part of a day's work. Although I was in the military, I never was hardened to the flight of life, although many who faced combat seem to have a different attitude toward the event. So maybe this part of caregiving won't take the toll on others that it took on me. Just know that it is part of the job and be prepared.

Another thing that concerned me was my own demise. We are all born terminal, so we can go at any time. I worried about something happening to me. Mother would not be able to handle a severe problem and I didn't have any idea what she would do. I made a key to the house available to Perry. He kept track of my coming and going and we stayed in touch so he would know that no problem existed. He and his wife, Jerri, were such a great help that I'll never be able to thank them enough. As you can see, nothing happened to me, but I had to have a plan in place. That's something that other caregivers should take seriously. There are so many things to consider besides the actual care of the afflicted person. As I said before…be prepared.

Chapter Nineteen

Another Angel Has Flown

Lucile Thomason Apperson
October 3, 1905 - March 7, 1994

It was March 7, 1994. The day was chilly and damp. Mother was taking her afternoon nap that usually lasted about two hours now. I had gone over to visit with Perry. We were sitting on his enclosed back porch around four o'clock. I saw my cousin Virginia drive up and park in front of the house. I went in the back door and let her in the front door. We exchanged our usual niceties and I told Virginia that I would go get Mother up.

The time had come. I went through that dreaded bedroom door and Mother appeared lifeless. It looked as though she had tried to get up because one leg was off the side of the bed. I called Virginia and we tried to awaken Mother, to no avail. Again my prayers had been answered: someone was with me at this very traumatic moment. It turned out that although Mother had lived for many years in the grip of Alzheimer's disease, it didn't take her. The death certificate says that coronary artery disease was the culprit.

I called Perry. He came right over with a stiff drink for me in one hand and his emergency phone book in the other. He had been a rescue squad member for years and knew the procedure by heart. He seated me on the couch and got Virginia situated in a chair. In no time at all he had made all the necessary calls. A steady stream of police, fire and rescue personnel started coming in the front door. I have never seen so many uniforms in one place since I was discharged from the Air Force.

I still cannot understand why it took half of the county in uniform to take care of the death of an eighty-eight-year-old lady. They would go into the bedroom and then back into the front yard and back into the house again. It was very upsetting to me. I was questioned by several of the sheriff's deputies and felt as if I were under suspicion of some wrongdoing.

Finally the Funeral Director arrived and removed Mother. At long last, the crowd started to subside. Virginia and Perry had gone home, and I was alone. Reality set in. In a very short time, my life had taken a sudden change and I was once again faced with the unknown. I spent a very restless night knowing that I had many things to take care of. I wasn't sure what to do next.

Being the fastidious lady she was, Mother had already made arrangements with the local funeral home for her cremation. All I had to do was some final paperwork. The Funeral Director was very helpful and gave me much needed guidance. Mother also had a simple will leaving me everything after any outstanding debt was paid. And she had everything in both of our names, so the house automatically reverted to me. In the face of it all, she had done her homework before she became afflicted and made my life so much easier.

Of course I would sell the house. My true home was in Florida and back I would go as soon as the loose ends were tied up. Things were working out and I was feeling quite a bit more relieved. But that bedroom door still haunted me...now for another reason!

Mother wanted for her ashes to be placed next to my father in my Granddaddy and Grandmother's burial plot in South Hill. She had bought a double headstone when Daddy passed and had it engraved with everything but her date of death. My cousin Carolyn took care of that last detail. Again, I don't know what I would have done without family. Mother was adamant that there be no service. She said that she didn't want people grieving over her passing. She would be in a better place and would rest easier without knowing that she was making people feel bad. She was definitely a piece of work! The Funeral Director suggested that I take the cremated remains on up to the burial plot and save some money. It would have been money in his pocket, so I am grateful for his honesty. I got my Aunt Hazel and cousins Carolyn and Phyllis to go with me.

Phyllis was driving and we were chattering together as we usually did as we went on to the Interstate highway. Not paying attention as we should have, we passed the South Hill exit and had to go to the next exit to turn around. As luck would have it, the sign said Bracey! Mother had taken her last trip to Bracey and didn't even know it. After all that joking when she used to check her watch for the bus to Bracey, the trip came true, even if it wasn't on a bus!

I had written a simple poem when Mother passed and had printed copies for all present. The service consisted simply of us reading the poem quietly to ourselves and leaving Mother and Daddy to continue where they had left off after 48 years of marriage. May they rest in peace.

On the next page is the poem that honored her. I had not only lost a mother, but one of the best friends a person could have...

Another Angel Has Flown

Thank you, God, for the loan of my mother
She touched my life as did no other.
With her simple wisdom and her gentle smile
She always went that extra mile.

This lady of grace is now at your side
With no Earthly sin for her to hide.
She served you on Earth and did her duty
By filling our lives with simple beauty.

My mother believed it was more blessed to give
And always tried to live and let live.
She saw your work as a marvelous thing
And thrived on the beauty that each day did bring.

You blessed us, dear God, by letting us know
How easy it is when it's time to go.
By your tender hand you spared the pain
And took this angel back again.

Thank you, God, for the loan of my mother
She touched my life as did no other.
Another angel has gracefully flown
To the kingdom of heaven and is near your throne.

In Memoriam

Appendix

Don't Take My Word For It

Here are some of the best references that I have been able to find.

There is a plethora of information available about Alzheimer's... its symptoms, treatment, caring for victims, and possibly even preventing the disease. I have included some of the best references that I have found. There is even more in your library or favorite bookstore. Also, the Internet is loaded with extremely worthwhile information. For the computer user, I have created a website where you can go to all three leading bookstores on the Internet or search the web for free information. Just point your browser to:
http://www.addsales.com/MyMothersKeeper/

Helpful addresses and phone numbers

Administration on Aging
Department of Health and Human Services
330 Independence AV, SW
Washington, DC 20201
Phone 202-619-1006   FAX 202-619-7586
Ask for Clinical Practice Guideline Number 19 " Recognition and Initial Assessment of Alzheimer's Disease and Related Dementias"

Elder Care Locator
800-667-1116

Alzheimer's Association
919 North Michigan AV, Suite 100
Chicago, IL 60611-1676
312-335-8700   800-272-3900 for information and local chapter referrals nationwide (24-hour telephone line)

Alzheimer's Disease Education and Referral Center
P.O. Box 8250
Silver Spring, MD 20907-8250
800-438-4380

References on the Internet

"Preparing To Be A Caregiver - Legal & Financial Issues for Alzheimer's - The Stages of Alzheimer's Disease"
http://www.alzheimers.com/

The Alzheimer's Association. The Alzheimer's Association is your source for information, support and assistance on issues related to Alzheimer's disease.   http://www.alz.org/

"Alzheimer's Disease: Caregivers Speak Out" provides the answers to many questions about Alzheimer's disease, early signs and symptoms, evaluation and research, as well as the emotional impact of Alzheimer's disease on our society.
http://www.chpublishers.com/

"Alzheimer's Disease Review" offers discussion of the latest advances in research on Alzheimer's disease and related disorders. http://www.coa.uky.edu/ADReview/

The Alzheimer's Disease Education and Referral (ADEAR) Center is a service of the National Institute on Aging (NIA). The NIA is one of the National Institutes of Health under the U.S. Department of Health and Human Services. http://www.alzheimers.org/

"The ALZHEIMER Page" is an educational service created and sponsored by the Washington University Alzheimer's Disease Research Center (ADRC) in St. Louis, Missouri. It is supported, in part, by a grant from the National Institute on Aging (NIA) (#AG05681). Opinions expressed are not necessarily those of the ADRC or NIA.
http://www.biostat.wustl.edu/alzheimer/

"Alzheimer's disease — What It Is" http://www.womenshealth-aging.org/alzheimers/alzheimers_what_it_is.htm

"The Alzheimer's Disease Cooperative Study" is a national consortium funded by the National Institute on Aging which conducts clinical trials for furthering the scope of clinical studies. http://www-alz.ucsd.edu/

"One Long-Awaited Step for Unveiling Alzheimer's Disease Secrets." http://www.meditopia.com/alzhome.html

Treatment and Management: A successful treatment plan should include several different components. It is important for caregivers to learn as much as possible about the illness and its effects on patients' behavior, ability to communicate and ability to accomplish tasks.
http://www.drkoop.com/conditions/alzheimers_disease/

Information about the Administration on Aging and its programs for the elderly, information about resources for practitioners who serve the aged, statistical information on the aging, and information for consumers (older persons and their families) including how to obtain services for senior citizens and electronic booklets on aging-related issues.

http://www.aoa.dhhs.gov/

Books sold in bookstores and on the Internet:

36 Hour Day : A Family Guide to Caring for Persons With Alzheimer's Disease, Related Dementing Illnesses, and Memory Loss in Later Life; Nancy L. MacE, et al, Paperback / Hardcover, 1999

Alzheimer: A Handbook for the Caretaker; Eileen Driskoll, Eileen Driscoll, Paperback, 1994

Alzheimer's: Another Opportunity to Love; Grayce B. Confer, Paperback, 1992

Alzheimer's & Dementia : Questions You Have...Answers You Need; Jennifer Hay, Paperback, 1996

Alzheimer's (A Caregiver's Day-By-Day Account); Robert V Rowe, Spiral-bound, 1998

Alzheimer's: A Complete Guide for Families and Loved Ones; Howard Gruetzner, Howard Greutzner, Paperback, 1997

Alzheimer's: Answers to Hard Questions for Families; James Lindemann Nelson, Hilde Lindemann Nelson, Paperback, 1997

Alzheimer's : Caring for Your Loved Ones, Caring for Yourself; Sharon Fish, Paperback, 1996

Alzheimer's; Hard Questions for Families: A Guide Through the Moral Morass of Caring for a Loved One with Alzheimer's; James Lindemann Nelson, Hilde Lindemann Nelson (Contributor), Hardcover, 1996

Alzheimer's: The Answers You Need; Helen D. Davies, Michael P. Jensen, Paperback, 1998

Alzheimer's: The Last Childhood; Carrie Knowles, Paperback, 1997

Alzheimer's Challenged & Conquered?; Louis Blank, Hardcover, 1996

The Alzheimer's Cope Book : The Complete Care Manual for Patients and Their Families; R.E. Markin, Paperback, 1992

Alzheimer's Disease; William Molloy (Contributor), et al, Paperback, 1998

Alzheimer's Disease; James E. Soukup, Hardcover, 1996

Alzheimer's Disease & the Dementias: An Alternative Perspective: Based on the Readings of Edgar Cayce; David, M.A. McMillin, Paperback, 1997

Alzheimer's Disease (Venture Books- Health and the Human Body Series); Elaine Landau, School & Library Binding, 1996

Alzheimer's Disease: A Guide for Families; Lenore S. Powell, Katie Courtice (Contributor), Paperback, 1993

Alzheimer's Disease: A Handbook for Caregivers; R. C. Hamdy(Editor), et al, Hardcover, 1997

Alzheimer's Disease: A Medical Companion; Alistair Burns, et al, Paperback, 1995

Alzheimer's Disease: Clinical and Treatment Perspectives; Neal R. Cutler(Editor), et al, Paperback, 1995

Alzheimer's Disease: Courage for Those Who Care; Martha O. Adams, Paperback, 1999

Alzheimer's Disease: Frequently Asked Questions: Making Sense of the Journey; Frena Gray Davidson, Frena Gray-Davidson, Hardcover, 1997-99

Alzheimer's Disease: Long Term Care; J. Edward Jackson (Editor), et al, Paperback, 1992

Alzheimer's Disease: Prevention, Intervention, and Treatment; Elwood Cohen, Paperback, 1999

Alzheimer's Disease : Questions and Answers; Paul S. Aisen, et al, Paperback, 1999

Alzheimer's Disease and Marriage: An Intimate Account (Clinical Nursing Research); Lore K. Wright, Paperback, Hardcover, 1993

Alzheimer's Disease Sourcebook : Basic Consumer Health Information About Alzheimer's Disease, Related Disorders, and Other Dementias (Health reference); Karen Bellenir(Editor), Hardcover, 1999

Alzheimer's Disease: Caregivers Speak Out; Pam Haisman, Paperback, 1998

Alzheimer's Early Stages: First Steps in Caring and Treatment; Daniel Kuhn, David A. Bennett, Paperback, 1999

Alzheimer's, a Love Story: One Year in My Husband's Journey; Ann Davidson, Hardcover, 1997

Alzheimer's: Making Sense of Suffering; Teresa R. Strecker, Paperback, 1997

Alzheimers, Finding the Words : A Communication Guide for Those Who Care; Harriet Hodgson, Harriet Hodgon, Paperback, 1995

The Alzheimer's Sourcebook for Caregivers: A Practical Guide for Getting Through the Day (Lowell House); Frena Gray Davidson, et al, Paperback, 1999

An Atlas of Alzheimer's Disease; M. Deleon, Hardcover, 1999

The Bad Daughter; Julie Hilden, Hardcover, 1998

The Best Friends Approach to Alzheimer's Care; Virginia Bell, David Troxel (Contributor), Paperback, 1996

Between Two Worlds: Special Moments of Alzheimers and Dementia; Ellen P. Young, Peter Rabins, Hardcover, 1999

Blue Moon (Life at Sixteen); Susan E. Kirby, Mary Stanton, Mass Market Paperback, 1997

Candle and Darkness: Current Research in Alzheimer's Disease; Joseph Rogers, Paperback, 1998

The Caregiver: A Life With Alzheimer's; Aaron Alterra, Hardcover, 1999

Caring for Maria : An Experience of Successfully Coping With Alzheimer's Disease; Bernard Heywood, Paperback, 1994

Caring for People With Alzheimer's Disease : A Training Manual for Direct Care Providers; Gayle Andresen, Paperback, 1995

Caring for the Alzheimer Patient : A Practical Guide (Golden Age Books); Raye Lynne Dippel(Editor), et al, Paperback, 1996

The Complete Guide to Alzheimer's-Proofing Your Home; Mark L. Warner, Hardcover, 1998

Coping When a Grandparent Has Alzheimer's Disease; Beth Wilkinson, Ruth C. Rosen (Editor), Library Binding, 1995

Coping With Alzheimer's: A Caregiver's Emotional Survival; Rose Oliver, Frances Bock (Contributor), Paperback, 1989

Coping With Alzheimer's: The Complete Care Manual for Patients and Their Families; R. E. Markin, Paperback, 1998

Coping With Alzheimer's Disease and Other Dementing Illnesses (Coping With Aging Series); Mary Norton Kindig, Molly Carnes, Paperback, 1993

Coping With Caring: Daily Reflection for Alzheimers Caregivers; Lyn Roche, Paperback, 1996

Day In, Day Out With Alzheimer's: Stress in Caregiving Relationships (Health, Society, and Policy; Karen A. Lyman,

Paperback, Hardcover, 1993

Delmar's Home Care for the Client With Alzheimer's; Jetta Lee Fuzy, Paperback, 1999

Dementia Units in Long-Term Care (The John Hopkins Series in Contemporary Medicine and Public Health; Philip D. Sloane (Editor), et al, Hardcover, 1991

Designing for Alzheimer's Disease: Strategies for Creating Better Care Environments (Wiley Series in Healthcare and Senior Living Design); Elizabeth C. Brawley, Hardcover, 1997

Developing Support Groups for Individuals With Early-Stage Alzheimer's Disease: Planning, Implementation, and Evaluation; Robyn Yale, Paperback, 1995

Doing Things : A Guide to Programming Activities for Persons With Alzheimer's Disease and Related Disorders; Jitka M. Zgola, Nancy L. Mace (Designer), Paperback, 1987

An Early Winter; Marion Dane Bauer, Hardcover, 1999

Elegy for Iris; John Bayley, Hardcover, 1999

Enhancing the Quality of Life in Advanced Dementia; Ladislav Volicer(Editor), Lisa Bloom-Charette (Editor), Hardcover, 1999

Facing Alzheimer's: Family Caregivers Speak; Patricia Brown Coughlan, Mass Market Paperback, 1993

Failure-Free Activities for the Alzheimer Patient : A Guidebook for Caregivers; Carmel B. Sheridan, Paperback, 1987

Fight Alzheimer's Naturally; Catherine Picoulin, et al, Paperback, 1999

Fireflies, Peach Pies & Lullabies; Nancy Cote(Illustrator), et al, School & Library Binding, 1995

Flowers for Mother: An A-Z Guide for Caregivers Coping With Alzheimer's Disease; Lynne, Selby, Hardcover, 1991

Forget-Me-Not : Caring for an Alzheimer Patient; Jan Charker, Paperback, 1994

Forgetting Whose We Are: Alzheimer's Disease and the Love of God; David Keck, Paperback, 1996

Gentlecare: Changing the Experience of Alzheimer's Disease; Moyra Jones, Paperback, 1999

Ginny: A Love Remembered; Bob Artley, Yasmin Khan, Hardcover, 1993

God Never Forgets : Faith, Hope, and Alzheimer's Disease; Donald K. McKim(Editor), Paperback, 1998

Gone Without a Trace; Marianne Dickerman Caldwell, Paperback, 1995

Grandma Jock & Christabelle; Barbara W. Casey, Paperback, 1995

Hannah's Heirs: The Quest for the Genetic Origins of Alzheimer's Disease; Daniel A. Pollen, Paperback, 1996

Harpo's Horrible Secret; Barbara Kelley, et al, Paperback, Library Binding, 1996

He Used to Be Somebody, 1995: A Journey into Alzheimer's Disease Through the Eyes of a Caregiver; Beverly Bigtree Murphy,, Paperback, 1995

Heavy Snow: My Father's Disappearance into Alzheimer's; John E. Haugse, Paperback, 1999

Home Care for People With Alzheimer's Disease (Aspen Patient Education Video Series); Aspen Reference Group, Hardcover, 1998

Home Care for People With Alzheimer's Disease: Activities of Daily Living—Booklet; Hardcover, 1995

How to Care for Aging Parents; Virginia Morris, Robert Butler, Paperback, 1999

I Want to Remember: A Son's Reflection on His Mother's Alzheimer Journey; David Dodson Gray, Paperback, 1993

I Can't Remember: Family Stories of Alzheimer's Disease; Esther Strauss Smoller, Kathleen O'Brien, Hardcover, 1997

If I Forget, You Remember; Carol Lynch Williams/ Paperback, Hardcover, 1998-99

In a Tangled Wood: An Alzheimer's Journey; Joyce Dyer, Ian Frazier, Paperback, 1996

In Sickness & in Health: Caring for a Loved One With Alzheimer's; William M. Grubbs, Paperback, 1996

In the Country of My Disease; Charles Pierce, Hardcover, 2000

Interventions for Alzheimer's Disease: A Caregiver's Complete Reference; Ruth M. Tappen, Paperback, 1997

Into That Good Night; Ron Rozelle, Hardcover, 1998

Is It Alzheimers?: What to Do When Loved Ones Can't Remember What They Should; Roger Granet, Eileen Fallon, Mass Market Paperback, 1998

Keeping Busy : A Handbook of Activities for Persons With Dementia; James R. Dowling, Nancy L. Mace, Paperback, 1995

Let's Talk About When Someone You Love Has Alzheimer's Disease; Elizabeth Weitzman, Library Binding, Paperback, 1997-98

Letters to My Aunt: An Alzheimer's Chronicle; Penny A. Petersen, Mass Market Paperback, 1997

Life With Charlie: Coping With an Alzheimer's Spouse or Other Dementia Patient and Keeping Your Sanity; Carol Heckmann-Owen, Paperback, 1992

Living in the Labyrinth: A Personal Journey Through the Maze of Alzheimer's; Diana Friel McGowin, Paperback, 1994

A Long Goodbye; Patti Davis, Hardcover, 1999

Mama Can't Remember Anymore: Care Management of Aging Parents and Loved Ones; Nancy Wexler, Paperback, 1997

The Memory Box; Mary Bahr, et al, Paperback, 1995

Men Giving Care : Reflections of Husbands and Sons (Garland Reference Library of Social Science, Vol 983); Phyllis Braudy Harris, Joyce Bichler, Hardcover, 1997

The Moral Challenge of Alzheimer Disease; Stephen G. Post, Hardcover, 1995

My Father Forgets; Lynn McAndrews, Paperback, 1991

The Mystery of Alzheimer's: A Guide for Carers; Elizabeth, Dr. Forsythe, Paperback, 1997

Nana's New Home: A Comforting Story Explainging Alzheimer's Disease to Children; Kristi Cargill, et al, Paperback, 1997

An Ocean of Time: Alzheimer's: Tales of Hope and Forgetting; Patrick Mathiasen, Hardcover, 1997

One Step at a Time; A Definitive Study of Alzheimer's Disease and a Practical Guide for Caregivers; Paperback, 1996

Painted Diaries: A Mother and Daughter's Experience Through Alzheimer's; Kim Howes Zabbia, Hardcover, 1996

Partial View: An Alzheimer's Journal; Cary Smith Henderson, et al, Paperback, 1998

The Positive Interactions Program of Activities for People With Alzheimer's Disease; Sylvia Nissenboim, Christine Vroman, Paperback, 1998

Profiles in Caregiving: The Unexpected Career; Carol S. Aneshensel, et al, Paperback, 1995

The Rakhma Story : Unconditional Love and Caring for People With Alzheimer's Disease and Dementia; Shirley Joy Shaw, Paperback, 1999

Research and Practice on Alzheimer's Disease: 1998 ; Bruno J., Md Vellas, J. L., MD Fitten, Hardcover, 1998

Safe Return Home: An Inspirational Book for Caregivers of Alzheimer's; Tom Batiuk, Chuck Ayers, Hardcover, 1998

Scar Tissue; Michael Ignatieff, Hardcover, 1994

Secret Waters (Womens Poetry Ser); Linda C. Brown, Sue Grimshaw (Illustrator), Paperback, 1997
Show Me the Way to Go Home; Larry Rose, Paperback, 1995

Speaking Our Minds: Personal Reflections from Individuals With Alzheimer's; Lisa Snyder, LCSW, Hardcover, 1999

Stress Effects on Family Caregivers of Alzheimer's Patients: Research and Interventions; Enid Light(Editor), et al, Hardcover, 1994

Stress Reduction for Caregivers; Anne Katz, et al, Paperback, 1999

Successful Communication With Alzheimer's Disease Patients: An In-Service Training Manual; Mary Jo Santo Pietro, et al, Paperback, 1997

Surviving Alzheimer's: A Guide for Families (Caregivers); Florian Raymond, Paperback, 1994

Tales from My Teachers on the Alzheimer's Unit: Poems; Sue Silvermarie, Andi McKenna (Photographer), Paperback, 1996

Tangled Minds; Muriel R. Gillick, Muriel Gallick, Paperback, 1999

Therapeutic Activities With Persons Disabled by Alzheimer's Disease and Related Disorders; Bowlby/ Paperback, 1998

Through My Eyes : A One-On-One Guide for Those Who Care for Loved Ones With Alzheimer's Disease; Shirley Anne Clayton, Paperback, 1997

Through the Wilderness of Alzheimer's: A Guide in Two Voices; Robert Simpson, Anne Simpson, Hardcover, 1999

A Time for Alzheimers; Florence Baurys, Paperback, 1998

The Validation Breakthrough: Simple Techniques for Communicating With People With 'Alzheimer's-Type Dementia'; Naomi Feil, Paperback, 1994

A Vow to Cherish; Deborah Raney, Paperback, 1996

What You Need to Know About Alzheimer's; John J. Medina, Paperback, 1999

What's Wrong With Grandma? : A Family's Experience With Alzheimer's; Margaret Shawver, et al, Hardcover, 1996

When Alzheimer's Hits Home; Jo Danna, Paperback, 1995

When I Lay Her Down to Sleep; Ann Wright-Edwards, Mass Market Paperback, 1998

Where Did Mary Go?: A Loving Husband's Struggle With Alzheimer's (Golden Age Series); Frank A. Wall, Hardcover, 1996

"Where's my shoes?" My Father's Walk Through Alzheimer's; Brenda Avadian, Hardcover, 1999

Will I Be Next?: Bea Gorman's Life Story - The Terror of Living With Familial Alzheimer's Disease; Lois Bristow, Paperback,

1995

Your Name Is Hughes Hannibal Shanks: A Caregiver's Guide to Alzheimer's (Agendas for Aging); Lela Knox Shanks, Steven H. Zarit, Hardcover, Paperback, 1996 & 1999